MAXIMUM FITNESS

STEWART SMITH

MAXIMUM FITNESS

THE COMPLETE GUIDE TO CROSS TRAINING

CONTRIBUTIONS BY M. LAUREL CUTLIP, RD, LD
AND JAMES C. VILLEPIGUE, CPFT

HATHERLEIGH PRESS • NEW YORK
A GETFITNOW.COM BOOK

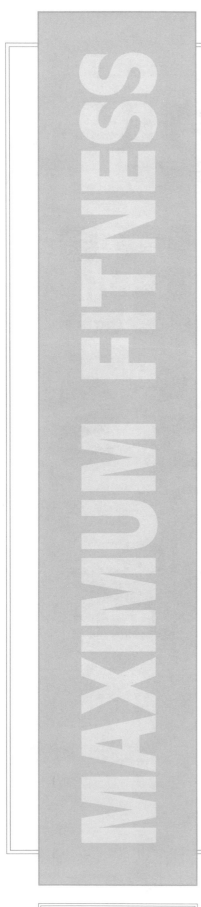

Maximum Fitness: The Complete Guide to Cross Training
A GETFITNOW.COM BOOK

Hatherleigh Press/Getfitnow.com Books
An Affiliate of W.W. Norton & Company, Inc.
5-22 46th Ave. Suite 200
Long Island City, NY 11101
1-800-528-2550

Visit our website: www.getfitnow.com

All Getfitnow.com titles are available for bulk purchase, special promotions, and premiums. For more information, please contact the manager of our Special Sales Department at 1-800-528-2550.

Library of Congress Cataloging-in-Publication Data
Smith, Stewart, 1969-
   Maximum fitness : the complete guide to cross training / Stewart Smith, contributions
   by M. Laurel Cutlip and James C. Villepigue.
      p. cm.
   ISBN 1-57826-060-4 (alk, paper)
   1. Physical fitness--Handbokks, manuals, etc. I. Cutlip, M. Laurel. II.
   Villepigue, James C. III. Title.
   GV481 .S6443 2001
   613.7'1--dc21
Cover design by Lisa Fyfe
Text design and composition by John Reinhardt Book Design
Photography by Peter Field Peck with Canon® cameras and lenses on Fuji® print and slide film

Printed in Canada on acid-free paper

10 9 8 7 6 5 4 3 2

Dedication

To those who purchased **The Complete Guide to Navy SEAL Fitness** and asked, "What do I do after completing this program?" Here is my answer: Thank you for your patience and good luck with **Maximum Fitness—The Complete Guide to Cross Training**.

I would also like to dedicate this book to Father Eric Hooge, who started working out with me when he was 80 pounds overweight and could not walk a mile without stopping. Within a year, he lost the 80 pounds and could run 15 miles non-stop. He dropped this weight to become a Navy Chaplain at the age of 52. Now Lt. Hooge is making an enormous impact on the lives of America's marines and sailors. Your dedication motivated me!

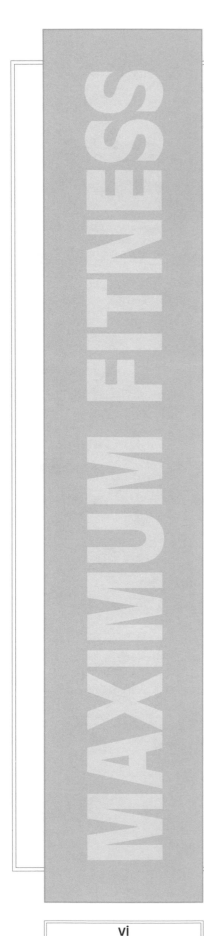

Definition of Cross Training

Cross training is an exercise program composed of several different activities to provide variety and reduce the risk of injury while improving overall fitness. A cross training program should include exercises such as walking, running, weight training, non-impact cardiovascular conditioning (such as biking, swimming, or roller blading) and flexibility. Cross training serves to maintain long-term interest and develop different muscle groups in a variety of ways.

Acknowledgments

I would like to thank James Villepigue, M. Laurel Cutlip, Tracy Tumminello, and Peter Field Peck for their contributions to the success of **Maximum Fitness,** helping turn this idea into a book.

Special thanks to my publisher and friend Andrew Flach for enabling me to stay in the fitness training business and write workouts that truly help people achieve healthy lifestyles. And to my wife, Denise, and daughter, Mary Elizabeth, who inspire me daily to work hard, play hard and have fun!

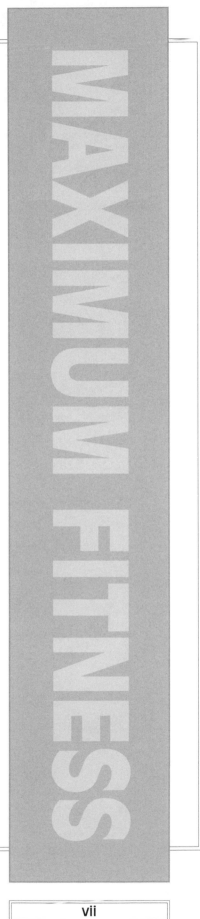

Contents

Introduction

Maximum Fitness—The Complete Guide to Cross Training is a culmination of almost every type of training—speed, endurance, strength, stamina, and flexibility—to help develop your cardiovascular system and burn fat. This book features a 52-week workout that splits the year into four quarters. Each quarter changes the focus of the training to give your muscles the most challenging workout of your life while resting your body throughout the year to prevent over-training.

Maximum Fitness encompasses all types of workout regimens for all types of athletes. Whether you want to cross train to break the monotony of your present program or wish to incorporate these workouts year round, the 52-Week Workout Program has something for everybody: a calisthenics, PT and stretching base; hardcore PT, running, biking, and swimming; weight training, PT, running, and swimming transition training; and weight training for strength. These various workout programs are divided into four 13-week segments. Each cycle builds upon the previous to prepare you for the next phase of the program.

If you have completed **The Complete Guide to Navy SEAL Fitness** (Hatherleigh Press, 1998) and want a change, this workout is for you. You will also find that the hardcore PT, run and swim cycle is even more challenging than **The Complete Guide to Navy SEAL Fitness** is. Likewise, if you have finished **The TV Watcher's Workout** (Hatherleigh Press, 1999) or **The Boot Camp Workout** (Hatherleigh Press, 1999), this 52-week workout can be your next step.

Maximum Fitness is perfect for every type of athlete: beginner, advanced, endurance, teen, and power lifters, as well as people who wish to lose or gain weight. You can benefit from any one of the four programs or utilize the entire cross training guide. This 52-week workout program builds a flexibility and calisthenics base and prepares you for more difficult calisthenics, endurance workouts and weight training. Core strength, flexibility, and endurance form the foundation to create a better athlete.

Cross training is the smartest way to train to become stronger, healthier and less susceptible to injury. Studies show that the ultimate cross trainers, triathletes, are injured much less frequently than marathon runners. In fact, over 50 percent of all runners are injured every year compared to approximately 25

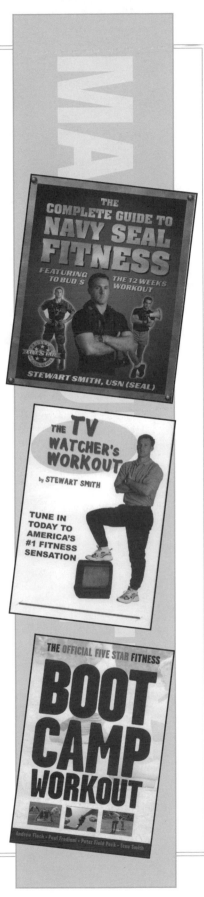

percent of triathletes. Power lifters who take a few months off from lifting heavy weights see larger gains in strength compared to those power lifters who "max out" year round. Everyone can benefit from cross training. Even the Navy SEALs utilize this type of cross-training program. They get lean and fast during the warmer months and beef up by lifting weights during the winter months to stay warm when diving in near-freezing water.

Personally, I enjoy breaking up my workouts into several different programs as featured in this book. I find that lifting weights for a 13-week cycle enables my joints to heal after several months of high-repetition calisthenics and miles of running and swimming every week. I also get my strength back during the first month of the power lifting cycle and build upon that strength, increasing my maximums every year. I typically add about ten pounds of muscle in the three months of the power lifting cycle and take it off again with the next hardcore PT cycle. I like doing this seasonally. In other words, I lift weights and gain weight during the fall and winter months—my hibernation phase. Then when spring begins, I run, PT, and swim again in order to lose the weight I gained and define it with the hardcore PT cycle. After a hardcore PT cycle, I like to mix a little weight lifting with my PT workouts with the weights/PT transition cycle just to prepare again for the power lifting phase in the fall/winter. I have been doing this type of cross training for over 10 years now and have had no injuries because of the workouts.

No matter who you are, this workout has it all—weight loss, weight gain, strength routines, speed and endurance programs, muscle stamina training, and more. Whether you aspire to join the military, are a young athlete, veteran exerciser, or even a beginner, this program will help you get to the next level of fitness. Start this 52-week workout at any phase you like and move onto the next cycle or repeat your current one. However, I would not recommend repeating the same phase more than two to three times in a row.

This program is designed to help you reach your goals- no matter what they may be. Maximum Fitness can be used for the following:

- Flexibility training
- Weight loss
- Weight gain
- Speed training
- Endurance training
- Muscle stamina
- Cardiovascular fitness
- Strength training

Concept of the 52-Week Workout

Give this workout three months and it will change the way you look and feel. Give it a year and it will change your life. Exercise should be as important a part of your daily activities as brushing your teeth or taking a shower. This book will help make exercise a constant part of your weekly schedule, no matter how busy you are. The special section on time-saver workouts can help you maintain your fitness level while traveling or if you are too busy for an entire routine. Additionally, workouts can become boring after several months of the same exercise machines, running or swimming routines. To avoid this phase of disinterest, and subsequent lack of motivation for beginners and advanced athletes alike, **Maximum Fitness** combines muscle strength, endurance and flexibility into one book. By cross training, you will not only retain interest while exercising, you stimulate different patterns of muscle and motor recruitment. Adapting to new stimuli causes the muscles to work harder by creating different types of resistance on the entire body. Exposing the body to a variety of exercises is the best workout plan for optimum muscular performance. Furthermore, you reduce the risk of injury by dividing your routine into several different workouts throughout the year.

IF YOU ARE A BEGINNER and have never sustained a lifestyle of fitness, you can begin your fitness journey with this one book. You will be amazed at how you look and feel in a few short weeks. You may be challenged by some of the routines in this book, but the object to getting started is doing what you can do comfortably. Starting will not be easy, but should not be extremely painful. If you follow the stretching week routine prior to beginning the first cycle of the program, you will be much less sore when you begin. The best workout program for every fitness level is one that incorporates cardiovascular exercise, flexibility training, resistance training and a healthy diet to give you the proper fuel to begin your fitness routine.

Each weekly program repeats twice until the 13th week of each quarter. This is for several reasons: 1) it enables you to try the workout again if you

Week #13 The Maximum Fitness Challenge

Week #13 should be avoided if you are a beginner. It is designed to have you reach momentary muscle failure, exerting your muscles to the max. Consequently, this causes your muscles to become stronger in an attempt to prevent future muscular failure. Beginners need to allow their muscles time to adapt to these intense workouts, without putting too much strain or force on the muscle fibers. Do what you can and if you cannot complete these workouts, keep trying. Remember, *something is better than nothing.* You will see results even if you are unable to complete the programs.

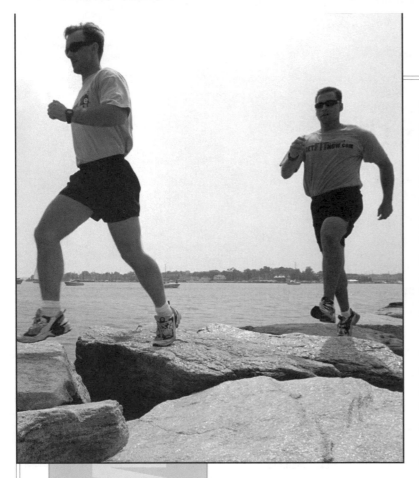

had any trouble with it the first time, 2) repeating the workout for two weeks allows the body time to get accustomed to the routine before changing it the following week, forcing the muscles to adapt to new stimuli, 3) it allows for a steady increase of difficulty as you approach the infamous *Week #13: The Maximum Fitness Challenge* The first 13-week program requires very little equipment. In fact, most of the exercises can be accomplished in your own living room. Stretching is strongly emphasized during the first 13 weeks. A short warm-up and stretch will begin each and every routine, followed by a longer cool down segment. A stretching routine is the most important exercise program you can do, *whether you are a beginner or a seasoned athlete.* However, stretching is often neglected for the sake of time. If I had only one exercise program to choose—out of running, swimming, biking, weight lifting, stretching, or calisthenics—it would have to be a flexibility program that utilizes basic Yoga positions. You will always feel better if you stretch properly than if you skip it. In fact, on days when you do not have time to exercise, try to squeeze in a ten-minute stretch to ease joints, muscles, tendons and ligaments. Many of the stretches in this book are adapted from **I Can't Believe It's Yoga** (Hatherleigh Press, 1999), which is one of the best books I have read to start a solid flexibility program.

SECOND PHASE

    THE SECOND PHASE is the hardcore run, swim, bike and PT program. This full-body program utilizes some of the same principles as **The Complete Guide to Navy SEAL Fitness**—upper body and lower body strength, cardiovascular endurance, speed, and agility. Most of these exercises are from the toughest training program in the world, U.S. Navy SEAL training. This type of hardcore calisthenics workout, combined with muscle isolation exercises and biking, form a safe and highly effective fitness routine. You might recognize some of these workouts from **The Complete Guide to Navy SEAL Fitness**; however, you will also notice that this book has new and improved workouts to take you to the next level of intensity.

THIRD PHASE

    THE THIRD PHASE is the weight and PT combination routine. The focus of phase three is less cardiovascular and more strength training. After the hardcore PT of phase two, this phase allows your joints to recuperate after months of high-repetition calisthenics and miles of joint-pounding running. There will be some calisthenics during this cycle, however, weight training will be slowly introduced throughout the weeks. Running will decrease, and biking and swimming will continue to keep up the cardiovascular fitness level gained during the phase two cycle.

THE FOURTH AND FINAL PHASE of this workout is the strength training program, featuring minimal cardiovascular training and more low-repetition, heavier weight training. You still briefly run, bike or swim to stay in cardiovascular shape, but the form of exercise will be your choice. Typically, this cycle is performed during the winter. Since most people prefer not to run long distances outdoors in the winter, you have the option of riding a stationary bike, swimming or cross-country skiing. The most important part of this phase is resting between sets of heavier weightlifting. Nonetheless, you still need to remain active during these rest periods. For example, after a set of heavy bench presses, take a two- or three-minute break before performing the next set, and slowly perform 30 to 40 abdominal exercises. This is a great way to pass the time between sets and will not effect your strength lifting heavier weights. There is a one-week "vacation" scheduled during the heavy lifting segment, immediately following the peak of the cycle, for your muscles to rest and repair. You will find that your strength will increase after a week of only stretching, light weights and cardiovascular training.

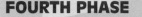

FOURTH PHASE

MAXIMUM

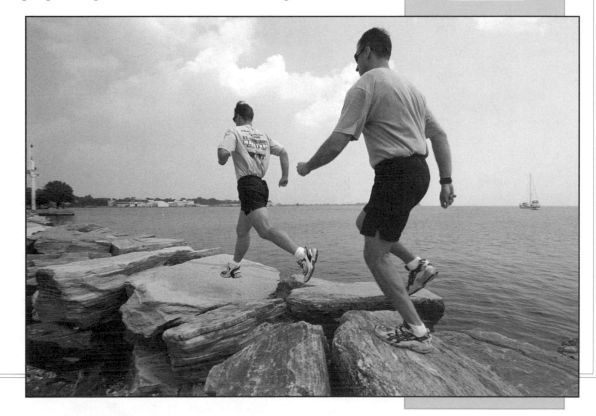

FLEXIBILITY: Beginning an Exercise Routine with a Stretching Program

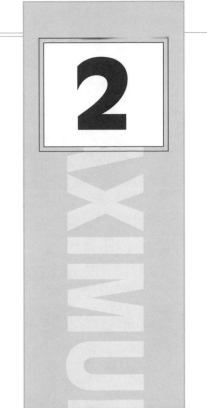

The Pre-Workout Stretch Week

This is the most important chapter in this book, especially for a beginner. By committing to a stretching routine, and increasing your water consumption, you will notice an enormous increase in flexibility and feel better than you have felt in years. By stretching for an entire week prior to beginning your exercise routine, you will substantially decrease soreness by as much as 50 to 75 percent when you begin your workout.

Although stretching does not require a lot of time, it does require consistency to see results. By following the program, you notice see a tremendous difference in flexibility in only a week. Most of my clients have a difficult time touching their toes, however after a few weeks of flexibility training, many are able to tie their shoes standing up for the first time in years.

Flexibility should be your primary goal before beginning any rigorous athletic activity. Increased flexibility has been proven to aid in blood circulation, prevent injuries, and increased speed and range of motion. A ten-minute stretching program after your workout will also reduce soreness the following day. That's right! The post-workout stretch is as essential to your workout as your pre-stretch routine. Soreness is cause by the production of lactic acid from maximum or near-maximum muscle exertion. Stretching aids in significantly reducing the amount of lactic acid that remains in your muscles after working out.

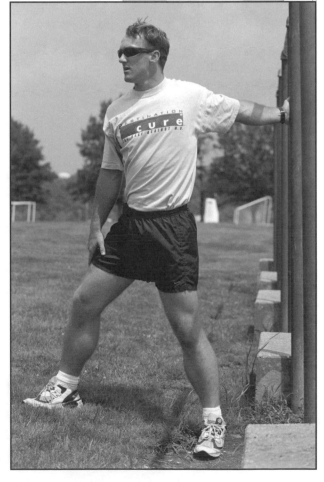

This simple head to toe static stretching program should be done following a brief exercise—such as a brisk walk, jog, or jumping jacks—to raise your heart rate, in order to increase blood flow throughout the body. Once you have started to break a sweat, you can begin stretching. This routine takes approximately 10 to 15 minutes, and should be performed twice a day for seven days. Anyone can find 15 minutes to stretch during the 24 hours in a day. Be diligent and commit to stretching each day. As long as you are drink-

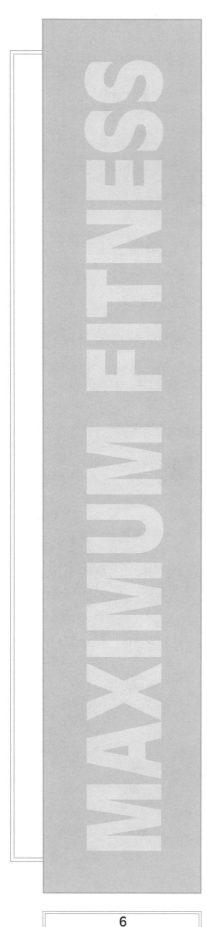

ing fluids and not exercising in extreme heat, I promise you will feel better after you have stretched. Perform each of these stretches for at least 20 seconds before and after your workout:

1. Neck Stretch
2. Arm Circles
3. Arm / Shoulder Stretch
4. Triceps / Back Stretch
5. Chest / Upper Back Stretch
6. Shoulder Shrugs
7. Cobra Ab Stretch
8. Knees to Chest
9. Thigh Stretch
10. Hamstring Stretch #1
11. Hamstring Stretch #2
12. Inner Thigh Side Stretch
13. ITB #1
14. ITB #2
15. Calf Stretch into Achilles Tendon Stretch

Descriptions of these stretches are listed in the pages ahead. The next few pages will illustrate some additional advanced forms of stretching to significantly help you with range of motion, strength, speed and agility. Do not begin stretching without a sufficient warm-up. You can suffer from severe injury by performing these stretches without properly preparing the muscles and joints. One of the best ways to ready the joints for advanced forms of exercises like sprinting, weight training and plyometrics is with dynamic stretching.

Dynamic Stretching

Dynamic stretching involves moving various parts of your body while gradually increasing both reach and speed of movement. Dynamic stretching consists of slow, controlled movements—such as leg swings, arm swings or torso twists—to gently extend the limit of your range of motion. Be careful not to bounce or "jerk" when performing these stretches.

In addition to improving dynamic flexibility, this type of stretching can be a useful part of a warm-up routine prior to an active or aerobic workout, such as boxing, sprinting or wrestling. Dynamic stretching exercises should be performed in sets of eight to twelve repetitions. Be sure to stop when you feel tired, since fatigued muscles are less flexible and will decrease the range of motion of your movements. Continuing to exercise when you are exhausted resets the muscle fibers at a reduced range of motion, which causes a loss of flexibility. Once you have attained a maximum range of motion for a joint in any direction, you should stop performing that movement during your workout. In the workouts to follow, you will use the following dynamic stretches:

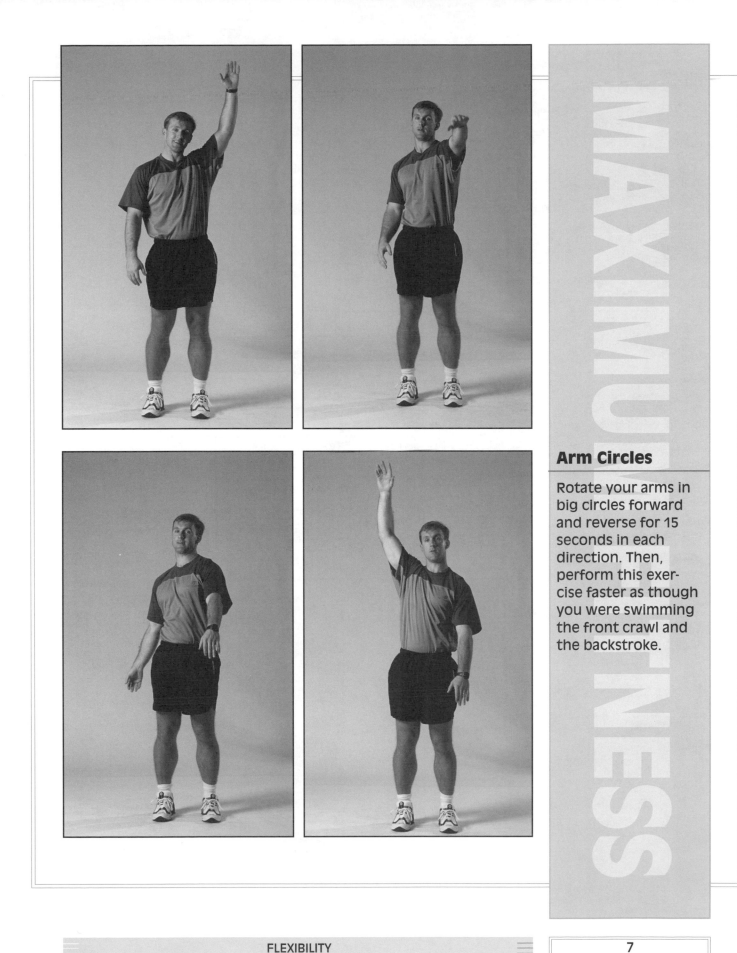

Arm Circles

Rotate your arms in big circles forward and reverse for 15 seconds in each direction. Then, perform this exercise faster as though you were swimming the front crawl and the backstroke.

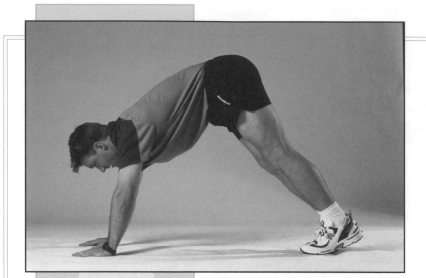

Butt Kickers

Start this stretch with both your hands and feet on the ground, and your butt raised in the air. Transfer all your weight to your hands momentarily as you try to kick your heels to your butt. Repeat 20 times.

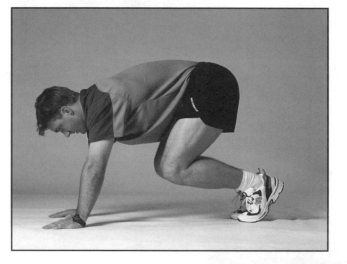

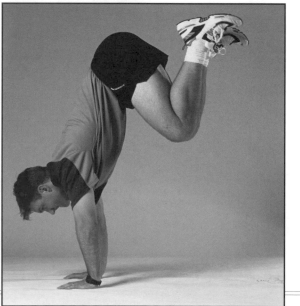

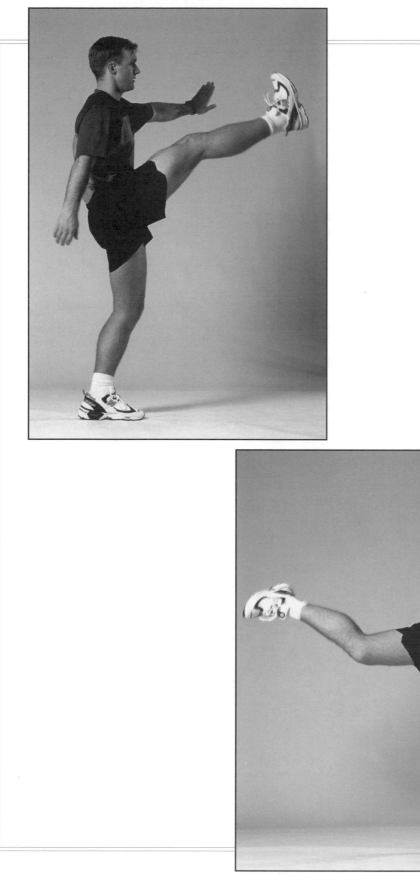

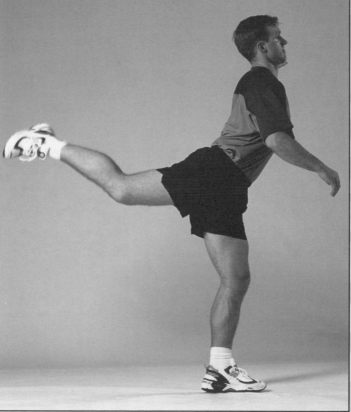

Leg Swings

Stand upright and hold onto something firm for support. Extend your leg from the hip joint forward and backward as far as your range of motion will allow. Perform 15 to 20 full rotations.

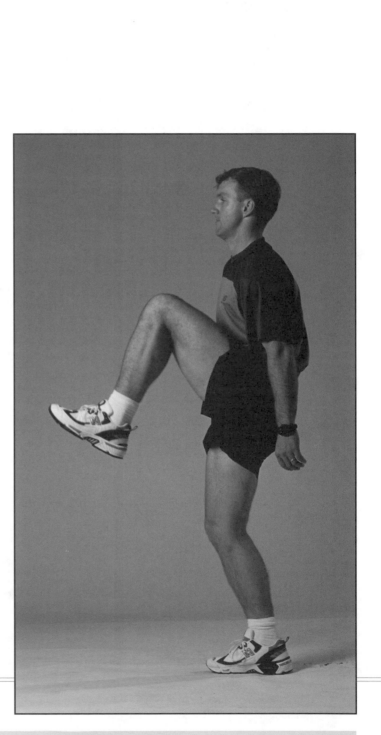

High Knee Lifts

As if you were running, lift your knees as high as possible (almost chest high) and skip across the floor. You can also perform this exercise in place if you do not have room to move forward. Repeat this movement 15 to 20 times per knee.

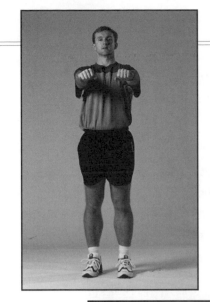

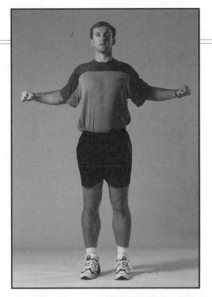

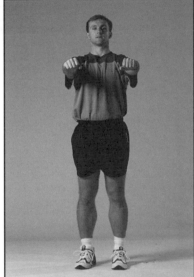

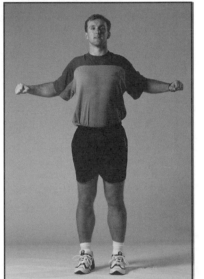

Press-Press-Fling

This is an old SEAL favorite. Extend your arms back as far as you can, keeping them parallel to the floor. After reaching back twice, pull back a third time and stretch your chest and arms as far as possible (without bouncing or jerking). This will prepare your arms and chest for push-ups and bench presses.

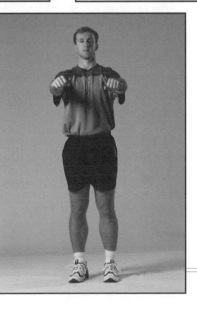

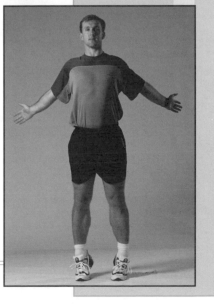

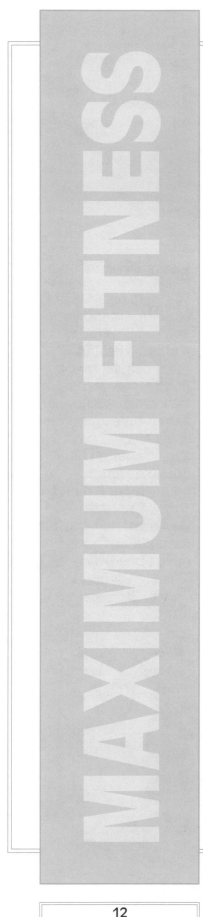

Stretching, Warm-up and Warm-down

Stretching is not simply a means of warming up, but is also part of the warm-down process. After a workout, the best way to reduce muscle fatigue and soreness—also know as DOMS (Delayed Onset Muscle Soreness)—is to perform a light warm-down stretching routine. This warm-down program is similar to the second half of your warm-up, but in the reverse order. Your stretching routine should consist of the following phases:

1. Five to ten minutes of a brief cardiovascular activity such as biking, running or swimming to adequately warm-up or warm-down the muscles.
2. Light or moderate dynamic stretches, such as arm circles or high leg lifts. Perform these light dynamic stretches until your heart rate slows to its normal rate and continue with a few relaxing static stretches.
3. Static stretching is the most common type of stretching. Hold a few stretches for 15 to 20 seconds each to slowly complete your workout. Do not bounce when performing these stretches and be sure to properly breathe—inhale deeply for three seconds, hold for three seconds, and fully exhale. Take two full breaths per stretch for optimal results.

Start your warm-down with approximately ten minutes of a sport-specific activity (only slightly more intense than your warm-up). Cardiovascular activity, followed by stretching, can reduce cramping, tightening and soreness in fatigued muscles. Furthermore, if you are still sore the next day, a light warm-up or warm-down is a great way to diminish remaining muscle tightness.

If you experience any pain or discomfort during, prior or after your stretching or workout routine, you need to try to identify the cause. Severe pain—particularly in the joints, ligaments or tendons—usually indicates a serious injury, and you may need to discontinue stretching and/or exercising until you have sufficiently recovered. See your doctor if the pain persists.

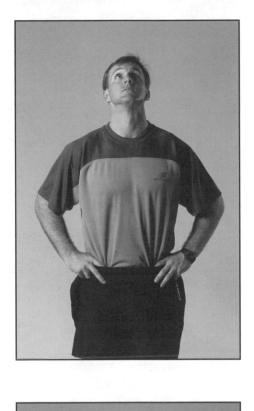

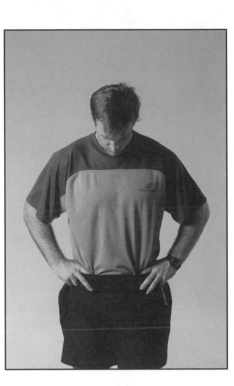

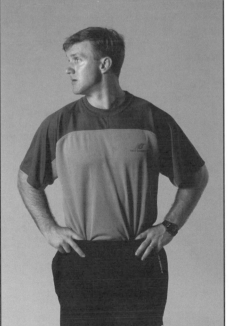

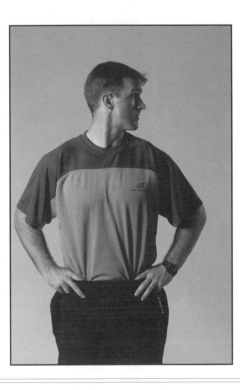

MAXIMUM

Neck Stretch

Slowly turn your head to the left, right, up and down, as though you were nodding "yes" and "no." Be careful not to raise, lower or rotate your neck too far. Neck injury can occur if this stretch is not performed in a slow and relaxed fashion.

FITNESS

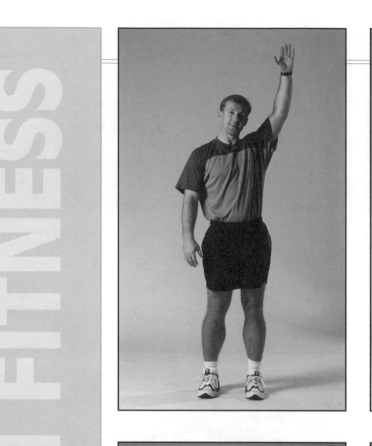

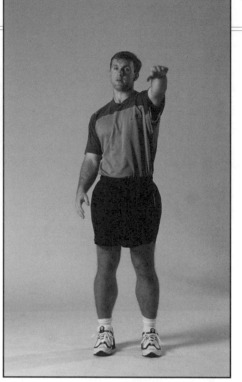

Arm Circles

Rotate your arms slowly in large circles forward and reverse for 15 seconds in each direction, as though you were swimming the backstroke and front crawl stroke.

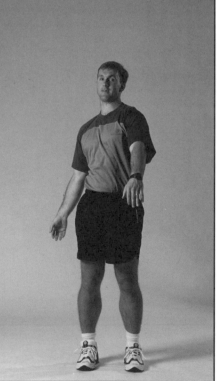

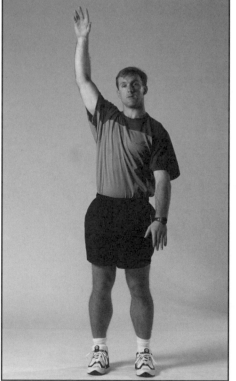

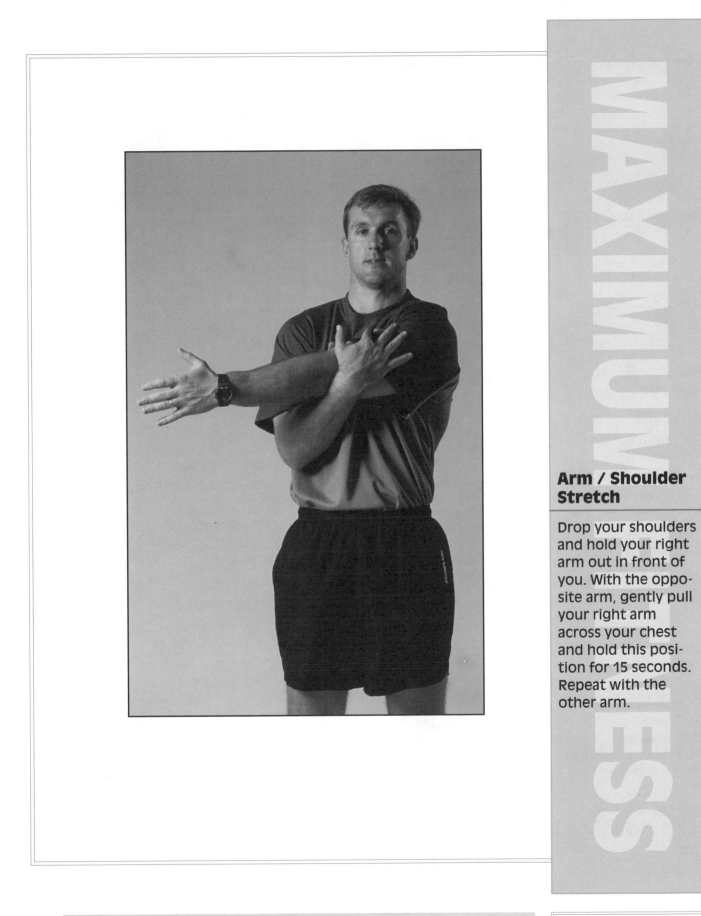

Arm / Shoulder Stretch

Drop your shoulders and hold your right arm out in front of you. With the opposite arm, gently pull your right arm across your chest and hold this position for 15 seconds. Repeat with the other arm.

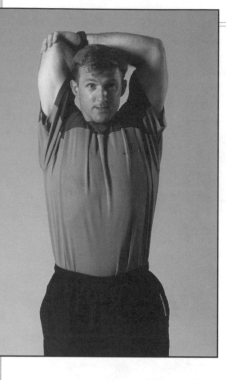

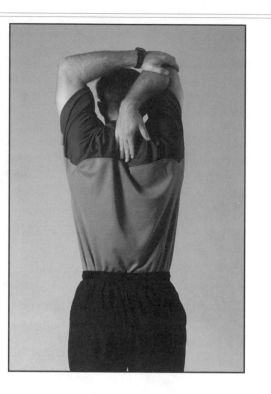

Triceps / Back Stretch

Place both arms over and behind your head. Grab your right elbow with your left hand and pull your elbow toward the opposite shoulder. Lean your torso in the direction of the pull. Repeat with the other arm.

This stretch not only prepares your arms for dumbbell triceps exercises, push-ups and dips, but also prepares the back muscles for pull-ups! This is a very important stretch for upper body exercises and swimming.

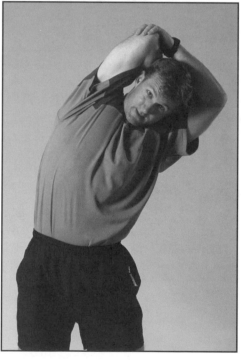

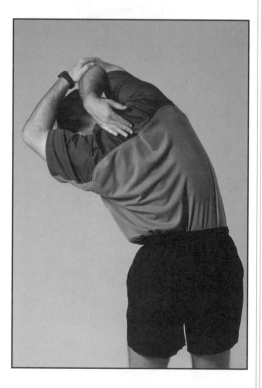

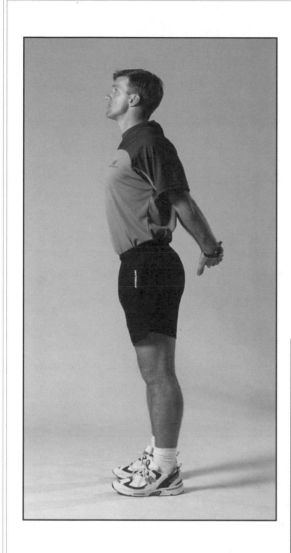

Chest / Upper Back Stretch

Stand with your arms extended and parallel to the floor. Slowly pull your elbows back as far as you can and interlock your fingers behind you. Squeeze your shoulder blades together and stick your chest out. Hold for 15 seconds. Then, round your back and bring your shoulders forward. This stretches the opposing muscle groups of the chest and the upper back.

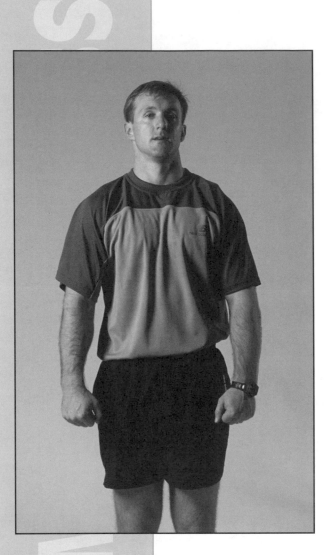

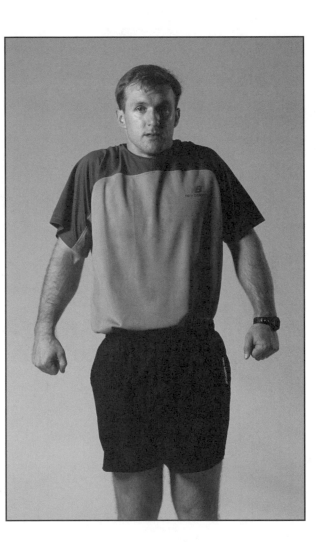

Shoulder Shrugs

Rotate your shoulders in small circles up and down in slow distinct movements, keeping your arms relaxed by your sides.

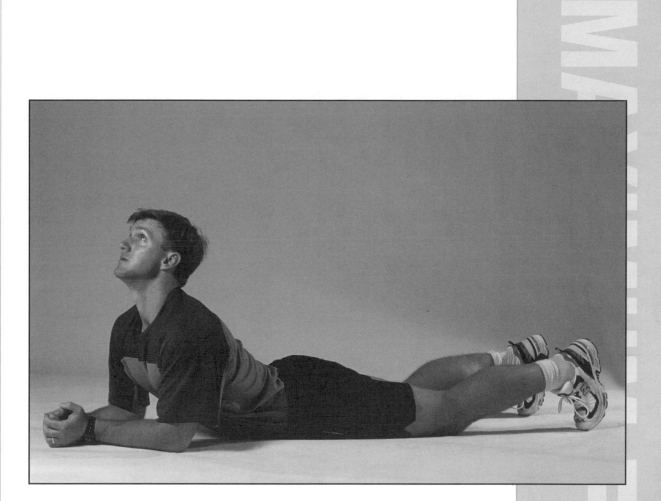

Cobra Ab Stretch

Lie on your stomach and push yourself up to your elbows, lifting your chest off the ground. Slowly lift your head and shoulders and look up at the sky or ceiling. Hold for 15 seconds and repeat two times.

Knees to Chest

Sit on your heels and bring your head as close to your knees as possible. Relax your chin to your chest and hold for ten seconds. This exercise helps stretch the upper back and the base of the neck.

This stretch can also be down lying on your back. Pull your knees to your stomach and hold for 20 seconds. You should perform this stretch before and after any abdominal exercise. Pull your legs over your head for a more intense lower back stretch.

As you may know, the lower back is the most commonly injured area of the body. Many lower back problems stem from inactivity, lack of flexibility, and improper lifting of heavy objects. Stretching and exercising your lower back will help prevent some of these injuries.

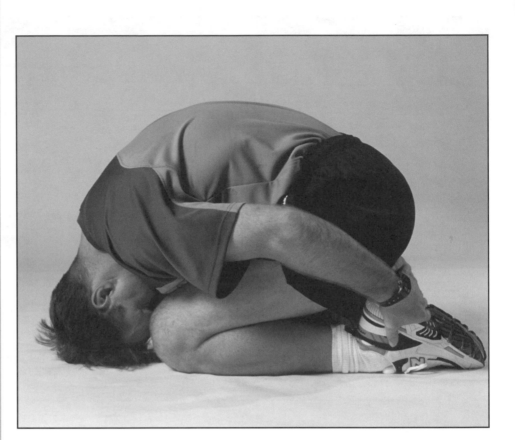

Thigh Stretch

Lie on your side, bend your knee and grab your foot at the ankle. Pull your heel to your butt and push your hips forward. Tighten your butt cheeks and keep your knees close together. Hold for 10 to 15 seconds and repeat with the other leg. This stretch can also be done standing.

Hamstring Stretch #1

From the standing or sitting position, bend forward at the waist and touch your toes. Keep your back straight and slightly bend your knees. You should feel this stretch in the back of your thighs.

MAXIMUM

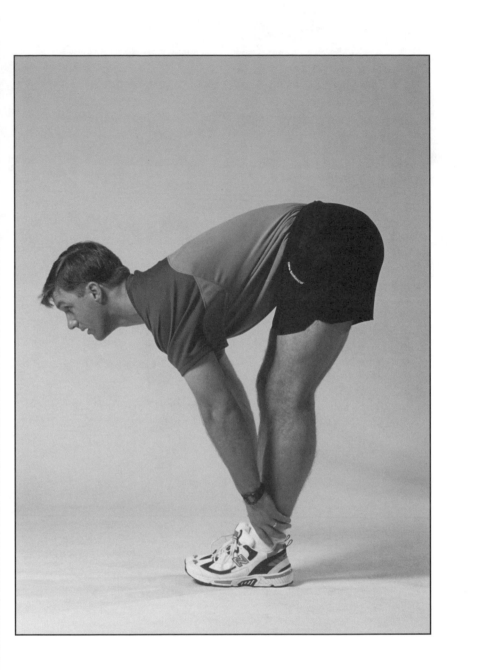

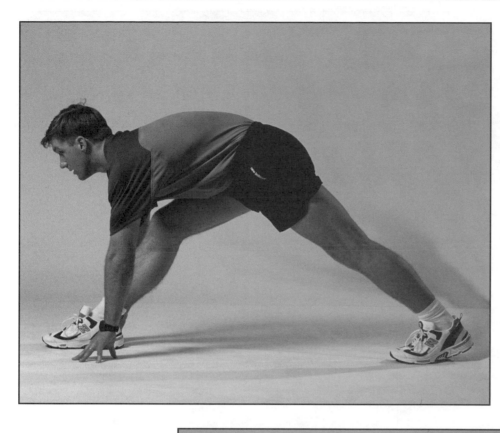

Hamstring Stretch #2 (Advanced)

Take a large step forward with one leg. Drop your chest to your knee and place your hands on the floor. Hold for ten seconds. Then, try to straighten your front leg for another ten seconds, keeping your hands on the floor.

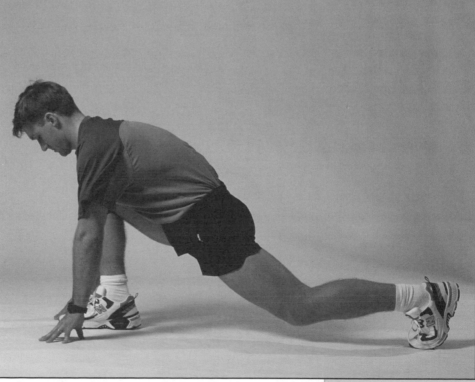

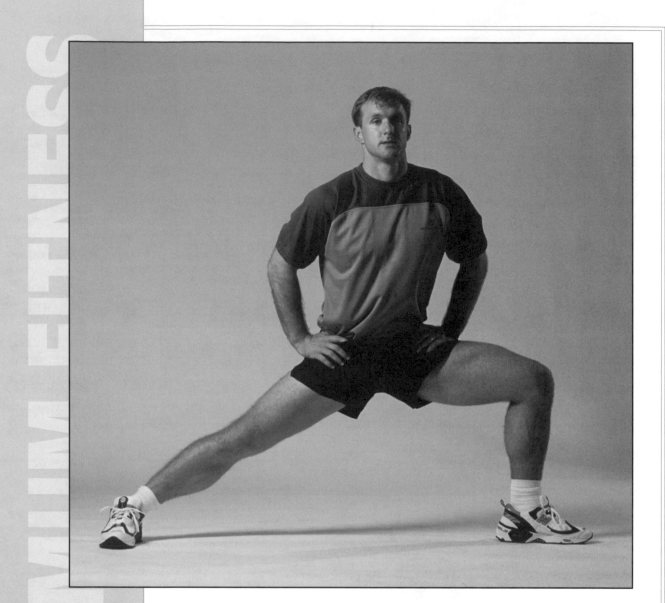

Inner Thigh Side Stretch

Stand with your legs spread and lean to the left/right. Keep the foot of the straightened leg pointing forward and the foot of the bent leg pointing in the direction the knee is bending.

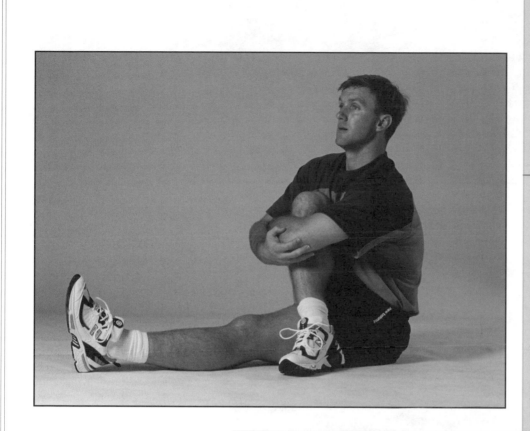

ITB Stretch #1

Sit on the floor with your legs straight in front of you. Bring one leg to your chest and bend it at the knee so that your foot is placed outside your opposite leg's thigh. Hold your knee for 15 seconds against your chest and repeat with the other leg.

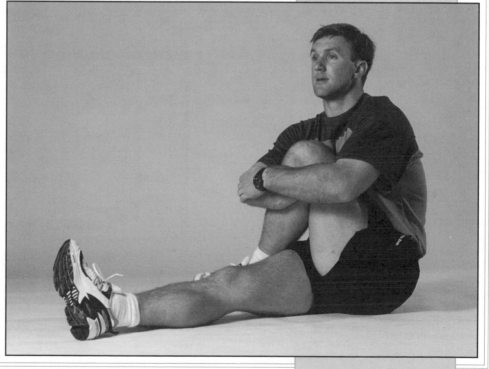

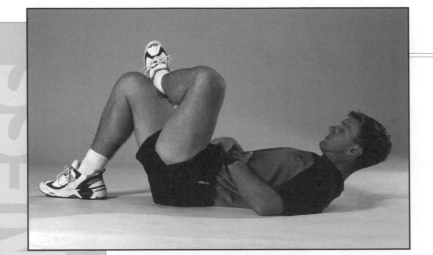

ITB Stretch #2

Lie on your back with your left leg crossed over your right leg. Bend your right leg and pull it toward you with both hands around the thigh or shin. Repeat with the other leg.

NOTE: Before and after running you should perform this stretch. This will help prevent common overuse injuries in the hips and knees.

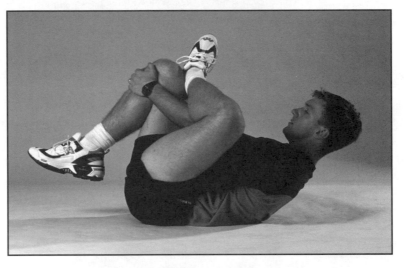

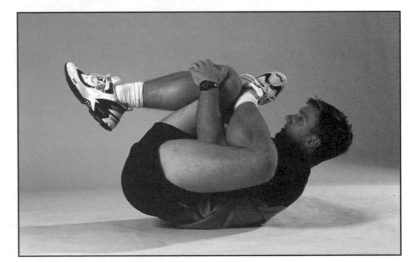

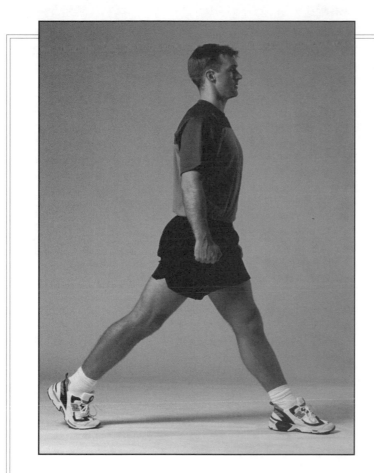

Calf Stretch into Achilles Tendon Stretch

Stand with one foot two to three feet in front of the other, with both feet pointing forward. Put most of your body weight on your back leg, stretching the calf muscle.

Now, bend the rear knee slightly. You should now feel the stretch in your heel. This stretch helps prevent Achilles tendonitis, a severe injury that will sideline most people for about four to six weeks.

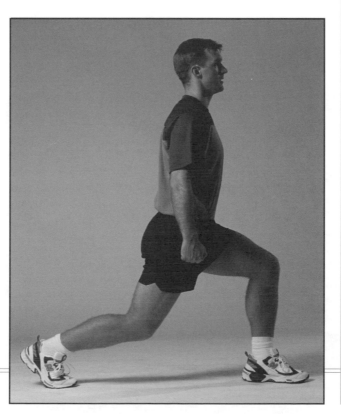

Explanation of PT and Weight Exercises

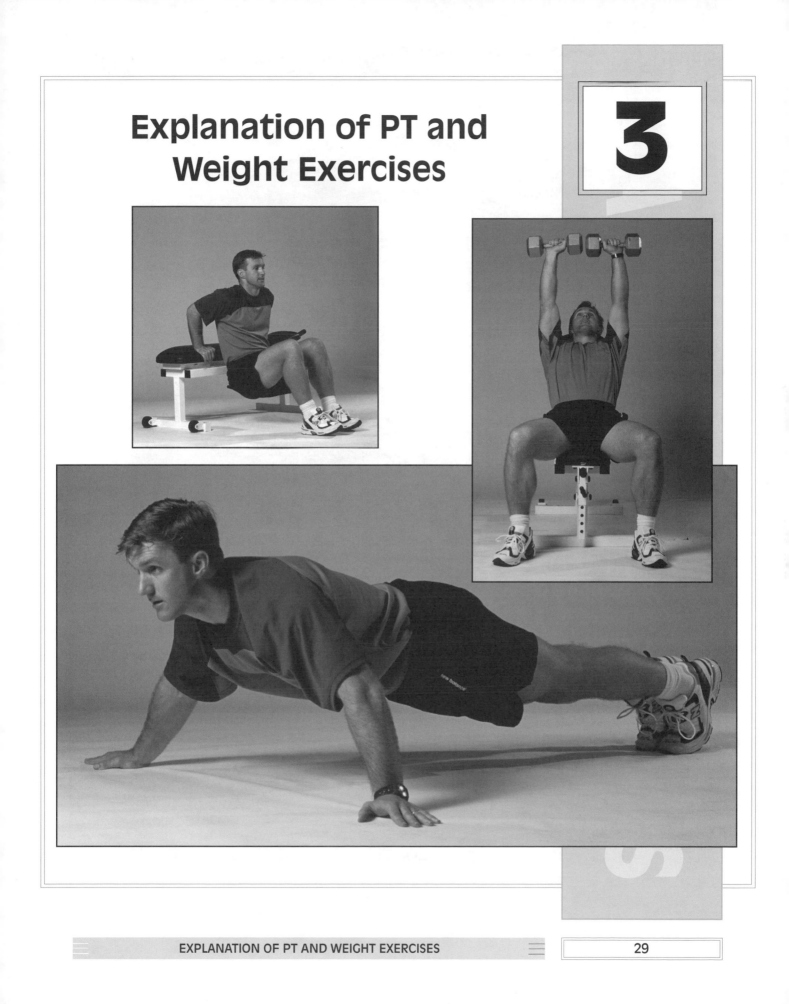

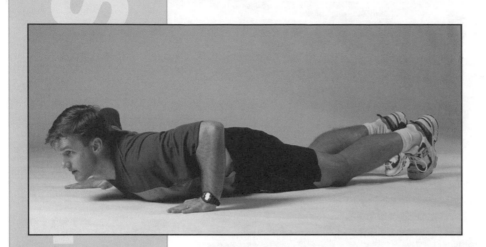

Regular Push-ups

Lie on the ground with your hands placed flat next to your chest, approximately shoulder width apart. Push yourself up by straightening your arms and keeping your back stiff. This exercise will build and firm your shoulders, arms, and chest.

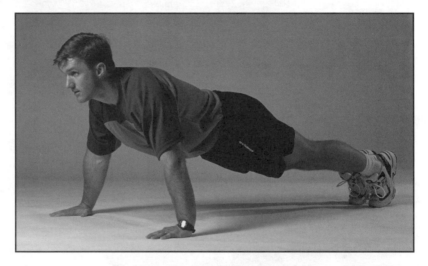

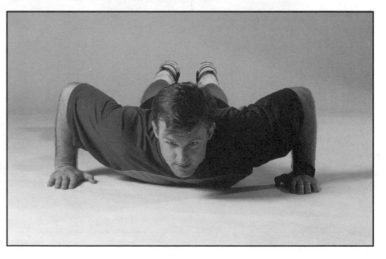

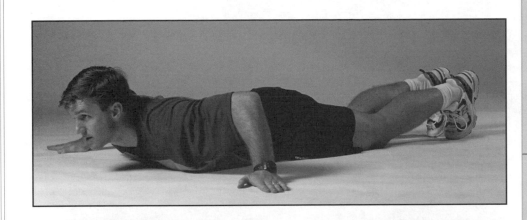

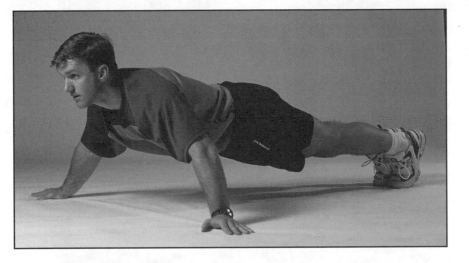

Wide Push-ups

From the same position as the regular push-up, place your hands about six to twelve inches away from your chest. Your hands should be greater than shoulder width apart. The slight change of arm distance changes the focus of what muscle are exercised. Now, you are building the chest more than your arms and shoulders.

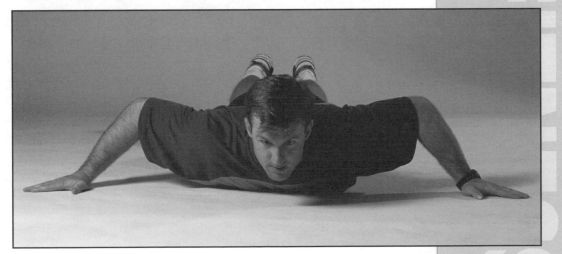

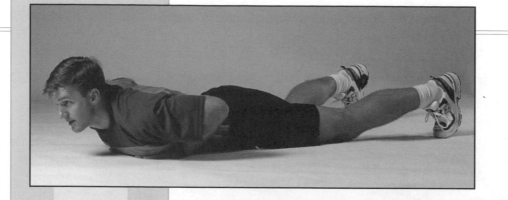

Triceps Push-ups

From the same position as the regular push-up, place your hands under your chest about one to two inches apart. Spread your legs to help with balance. This exercise will concentrate more on the triceps than the chest.

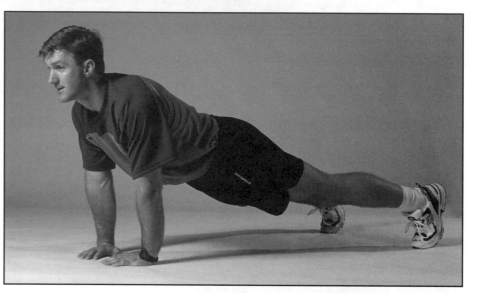

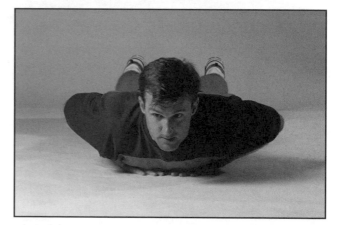

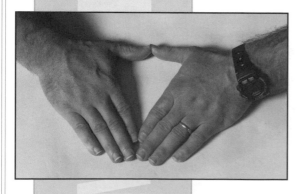

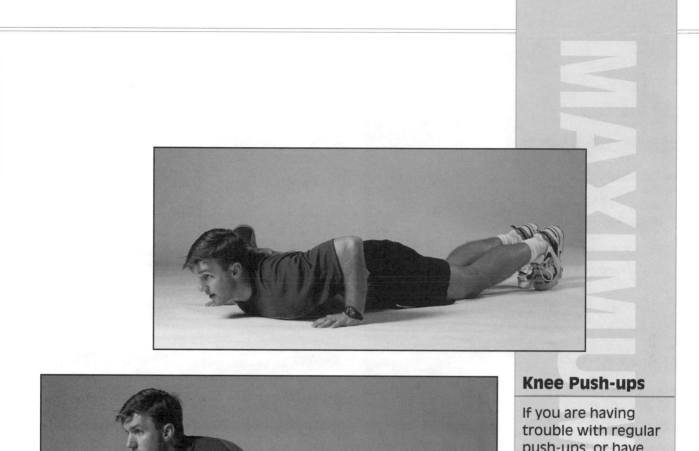

Knee Push-ups

If you are having trouble with regular push-ups, or have reached muscle fatigue in your push-up workout, you can resort to knee push-ups and receive the same muscular benefit. Lie on the ground. With your knees remaining on the ground, lift your body off the floor by straightening your arms and keeping your back stiff.

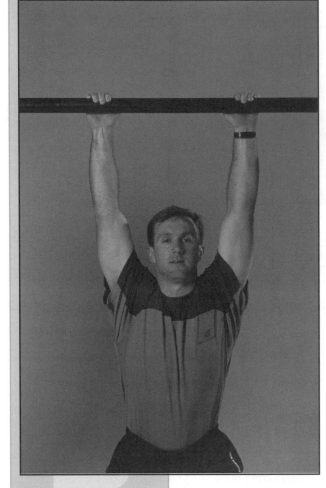

Regular Grip Pull-ups

Grab the pull-up bar with your hands placed approximately shoulder width apart and your palms facing away from you. Pull yourself upward until your chin is over the bar and complete the exercise by slowly returning to the hanging position.

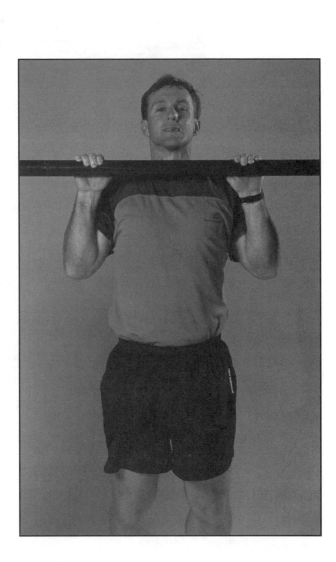

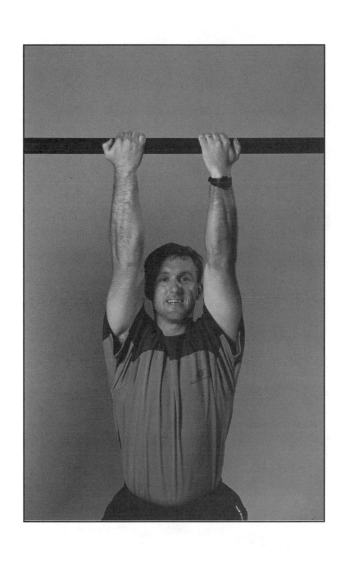

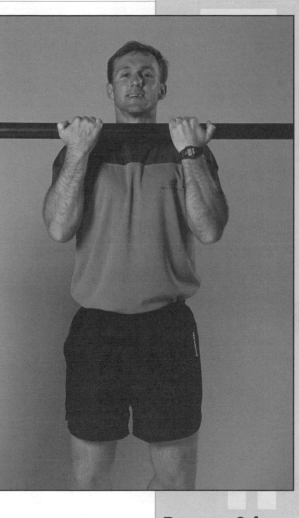

Reverse Grip Pull-ups

Grab the pull-up bar with your hands placed about two to three inches apart with your palms facing you. Pull yourself upward until your chin is over the bar and complete the exercise by slowly returning to the hanging position.

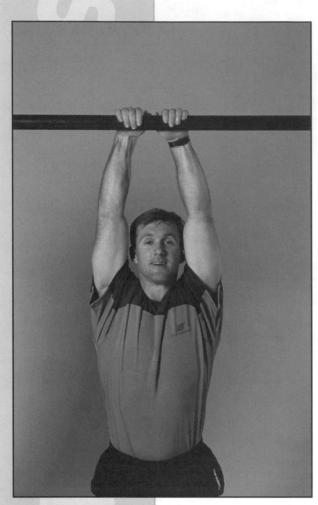

Close Grip Pull-ups

Grab the pull-up bar with your hands placed about an inch apart and your palms facing away from you. Pull yourself upward until your chin is over the bar and complete the exercise by slowly returning to the hanging position.

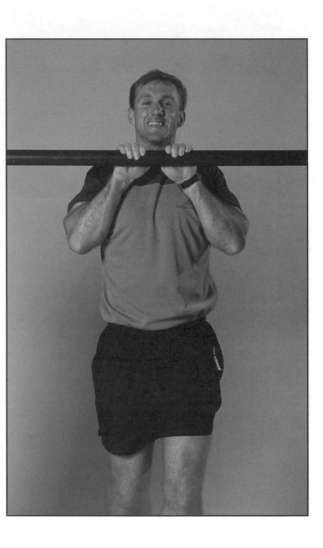

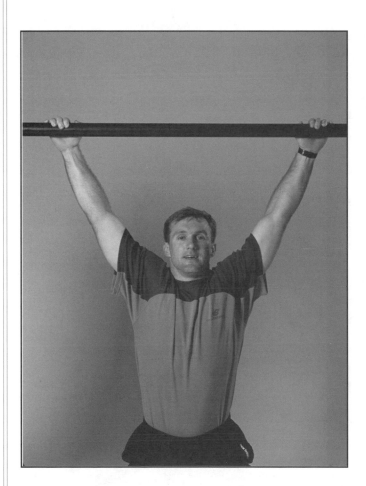

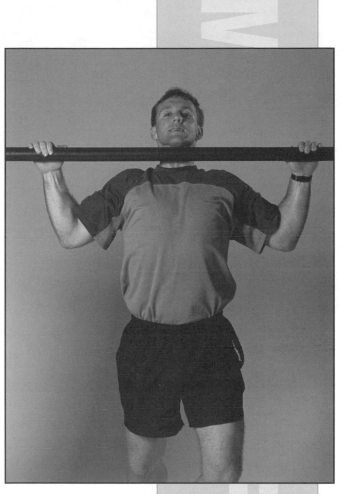

Wide Grip Pull-up

Grab the pull-up bar with your hands placed slightly wider than shoulder width apart and your palms facing away from you. Pull yourself upward until your chin is over the bar and complete the exercise by slowly returning to the hanging position.

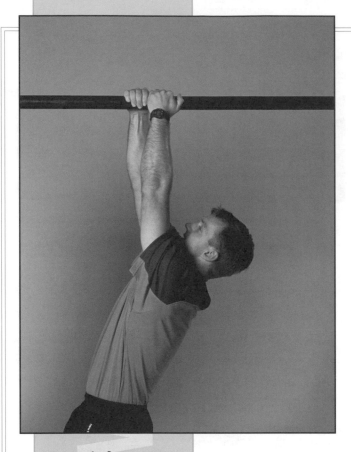

Mountain Climber Grip

Grab the pull-up bar with your hands placed about an inch apart and one palm facing away from you and the other facing you. Pull yourself upward until your shoulder touches the bar. Repeat on each side for a total of two pull-ups—one per shoulder.

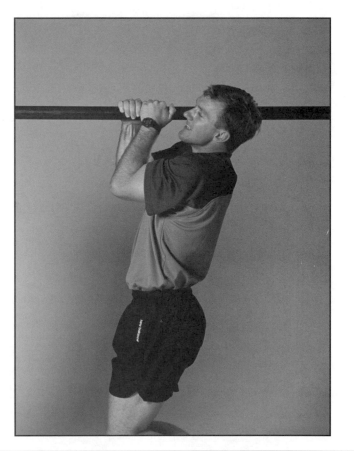

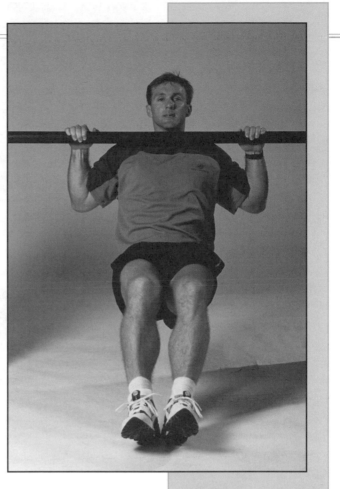

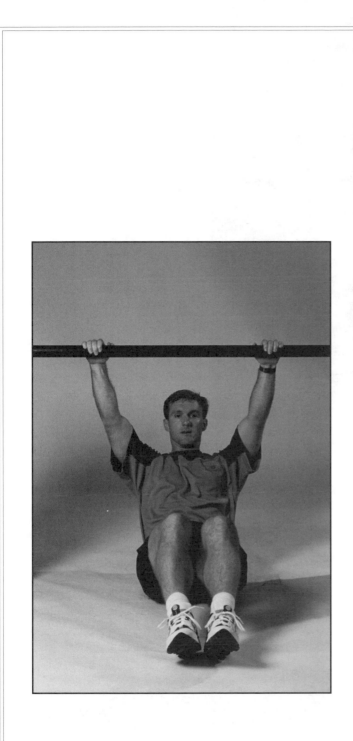

Assisted Pull-ups

Sit under a bar that is three to four feet off the ground and grab the bar with the regular grip. Straighten your back, hips and legs and pull yourself upward until your chest touches the bar. Repeat as required. *This is a great way to begin if you cannot do any pull-ups. This exercise can also be performed with parallel bars, which are used for dips.*

Negative
Pull-ups and Dips

If you cannot do any pull-ups, begin by doing negatives. Negatives are essentially half pull-ups. All you have to do is get your chin over the bar, by standing on a chair for instance. Then, slowly lower yourself all the way down, letting your fully extended arms hang from the bar. Resist gravity as much as you can—that is what makes this exercise tough. *Do not put your feet back on the chair.* Keep those feet up and fight gravity for a count of five seconds.

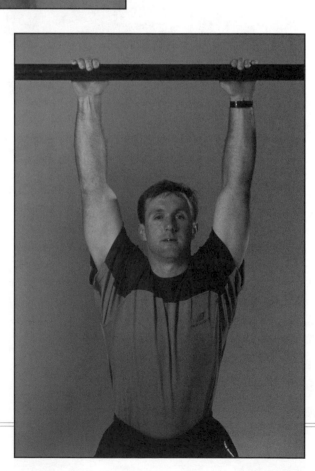

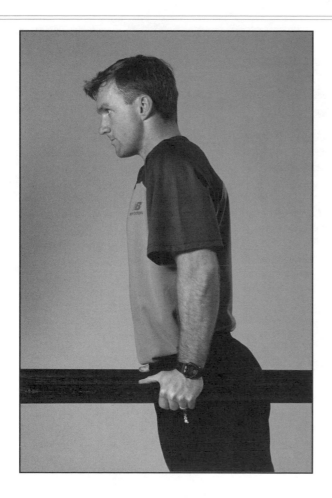

Parallel Bar Dips

Grab the bars with both hands and rest all of your weight on your arms and shoulders. Sound dangerous? It is! Do not perform these exercises with added weights, if you are a beginner, or if you have had a previous shoulder injury. Complete this exercise by lowering yourself until your elbows form a 90-degree angle and return to the upright position.

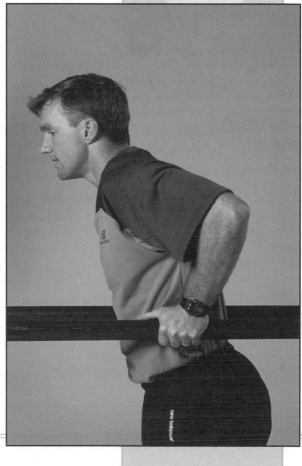

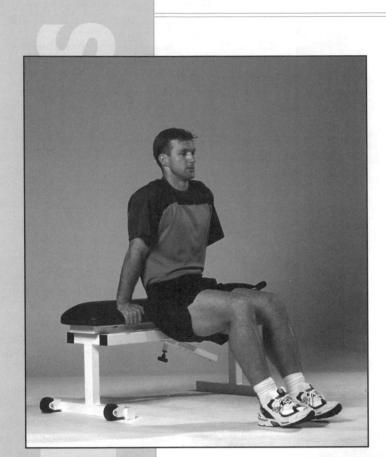

Bench Dips

Sit on a chair, bench or small table. Place your feet about three feet in front of you as you sit on the very edge of the seat. Now, grab the edge of the seat with your hands, lift up your butt, and lower yourself about four to five inches below the seat by bending your arms at the elbow. Straighten your arms and repeat.

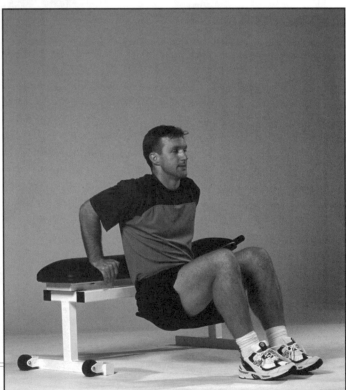

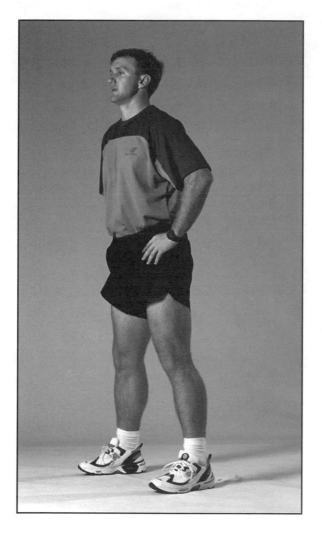

Squats

Keep your feet shoulder width apart. Drop your butt back as though sitting in a chair. Keep your heels on the ground and your knees over your ankles. Your shins should be near vertical at all times and your butt should extend backward. This exercise works the glutes, quadriceps, and hamstrings.

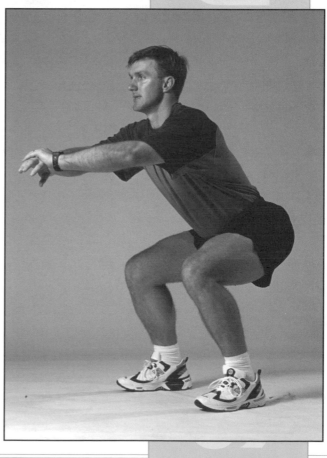

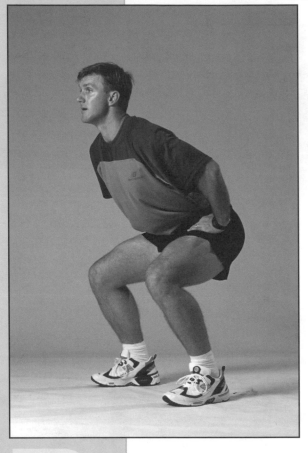

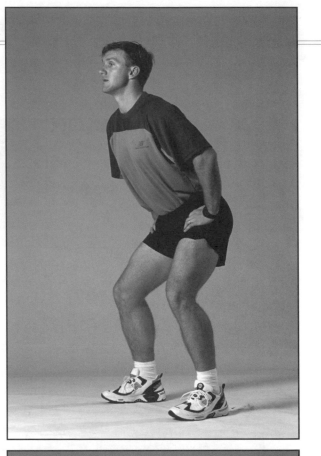

Half-Squats

Intensify your squat by doing half-squats. While in the full squat position, hold the pose and alternate up and down within a six-inch range of motion, similar to riding a horse.

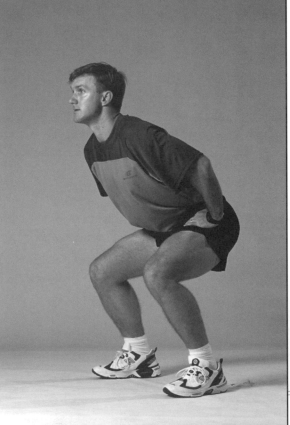

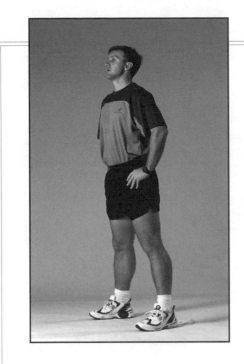

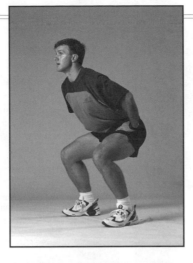

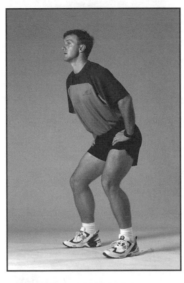

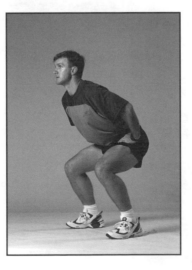

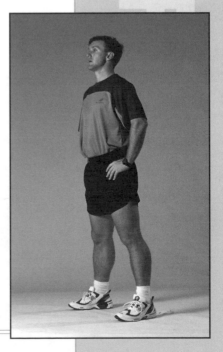

Four-Count Squats

1. Start by lowering to the full squat position,

2. lift half way,

3. drop back down to a full squat,

4. finish by returning to a standing position.

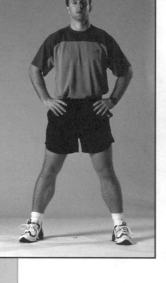

Side-Stepping Squats

From the full squat position, push upward as you shuffle your feet to the left or right. After each step, stop and do a full squat. You can alternate left and right steps if you do not have much room or you can do ten side squats to the left, then ten side squats to the right.

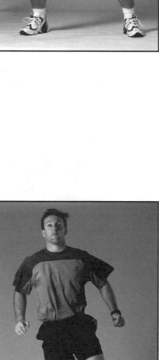

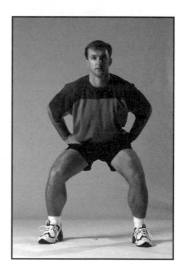

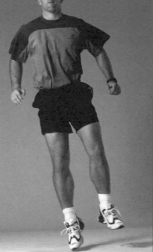

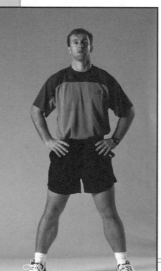

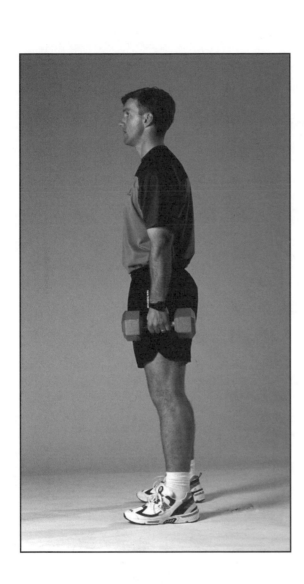

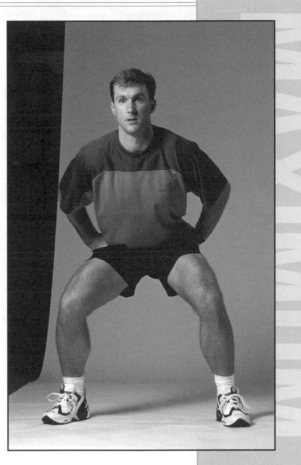

Squats With Weights

This exercise can be done with dumb-bells, carried outside your thighs, or with a barbell, placed just below your shoul-ders. Keep your back straight and look toward the ceiling. Lower your body until your thighs are approximately parallel to the floor, keeping your shins vertical.

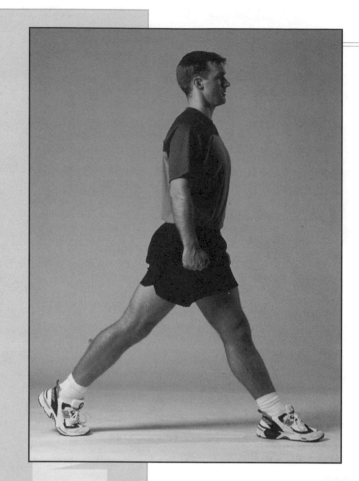

Walking Lunge

The lunge is a great leg exercise to develop shape and flexibility. Keep your chest up high and your stomach tight. Take a long step forward and drop your back knee toward the ground. Stand up on your forward leg, bringing your feet together and repeat with the other leg. Be careful your knee never extends past your foot. Muscles used: quadriceps, hamstrings, and glutes.

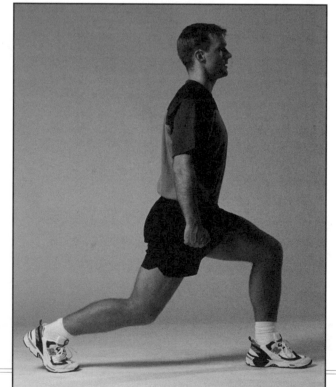

Stationary Lunge

Take a big step forward. Bend both knees and lower your body until your front thigh is approximately parallel to the floor. Slowly lift your body until your knees are straight, keeping your feet in the same position. If you have bad knees, either avoid this exercise or only drop halfway down.

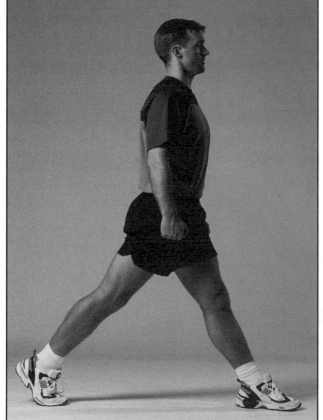

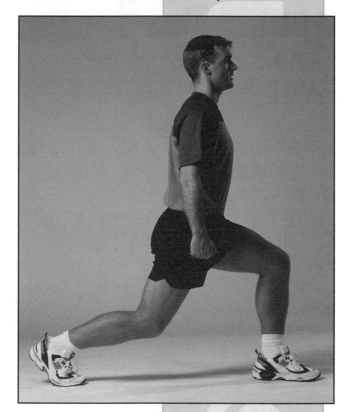

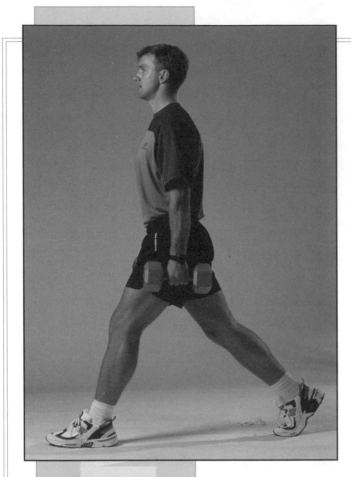

Lunge With Weights

Only the stationary lunge should be performed with weights, since it's easier on the knees than the walking lunge. Simply hold the weights at your side with your arms relaxed. Do at least ten lunges with each leg.

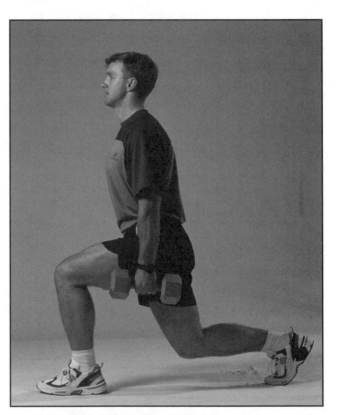

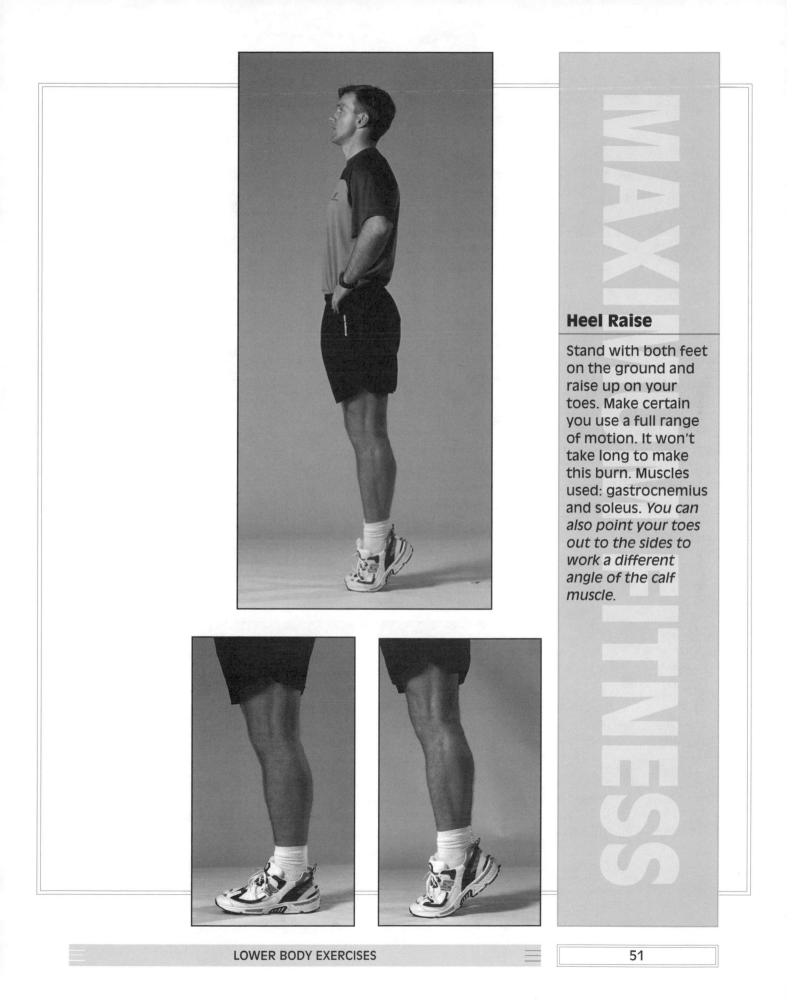

Heel Raise

Stand with both feet on the ground and raise up on your toes. Make certain you use a full range of motion. It won't take long to make this burn. Muscles used: gastrocnemius and soleus. *You can also point your toes out to the sides to work a different angle of the calf muscle.*

Bent Knee Heel Raise

As you lift your heel off the floor, bend your knees slightly. This will isolate the soleus—the muscle used for jumping high and starting sprints.

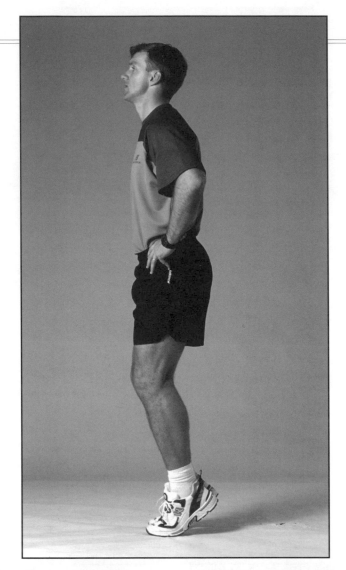

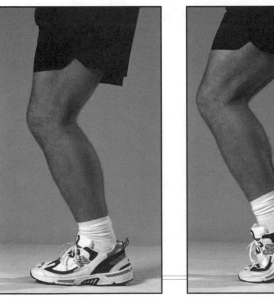

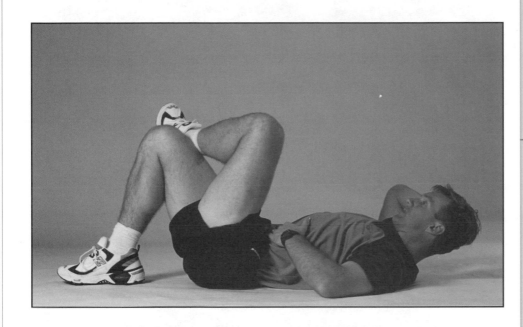

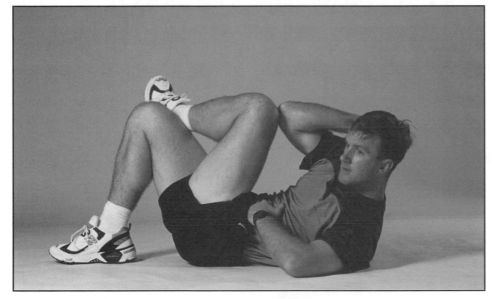

Right Elbow to Left Knee

Cross your left leg over your right leg. Flex your stomach and twist to bring your right elbow to your left knee.

When exercising the stomach muscles, make sure to exercise and stretch your back as well. The stomach and lower back muscles are opposing muscle groups. If one is much stronger than the other is, you can easily injure the weaker muscle group.

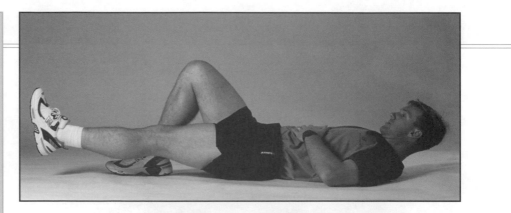

Leg Lever Version

Keeping your right leg bent with your foot flat on the floor, straighten your left leg and lift it toward the ceiling. Touch your right elbow to your left knee and relax your shoulders back to the resting position. Lower your leg six inches off the floor, keeping your leg straight. Muscles used: obliques, hip flexors, thighs, and hamstrings.

Avoid this exercise if you have had a previous lower back injury.

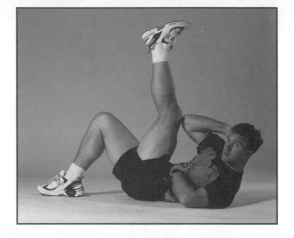

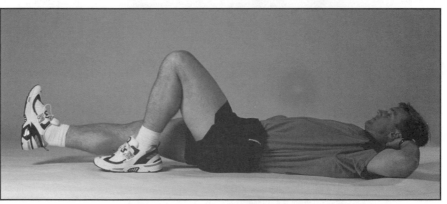

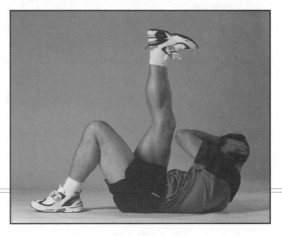

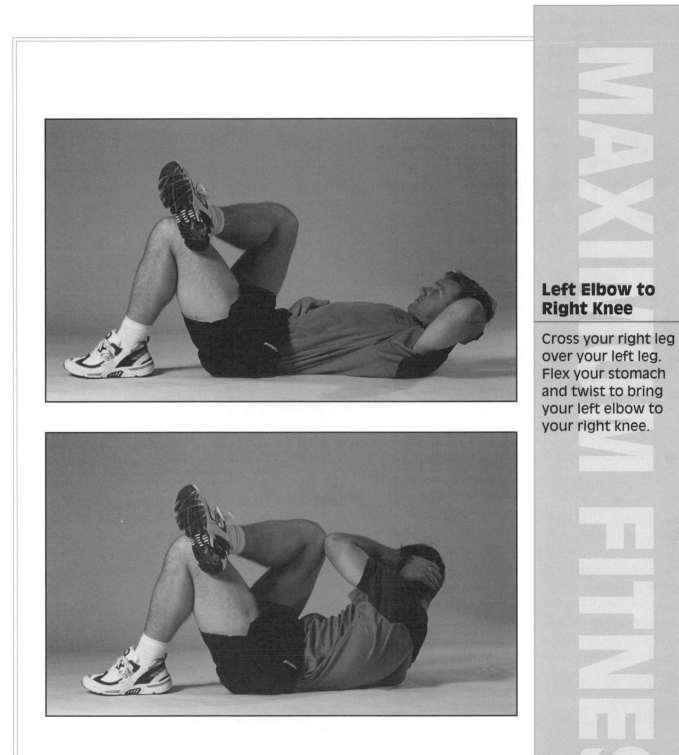

Left Elbow to Right Knee

Cross your right leg over your left leg. Flex your stomach and twist to bring your left elbow to your right knee.

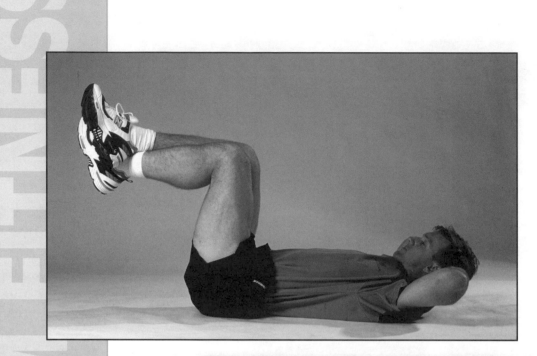

Reverse Crunch

In the same position as the regular crunch, lift your knees and butt toward your elbows. Leave your head and upper body flat on the ground. *Avoid this exercise if you have had a previous lower back injury.*

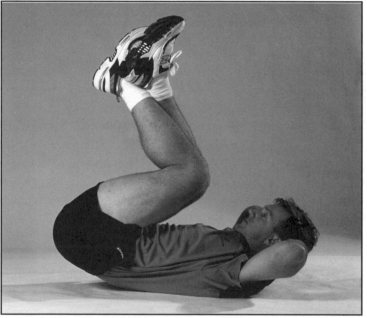

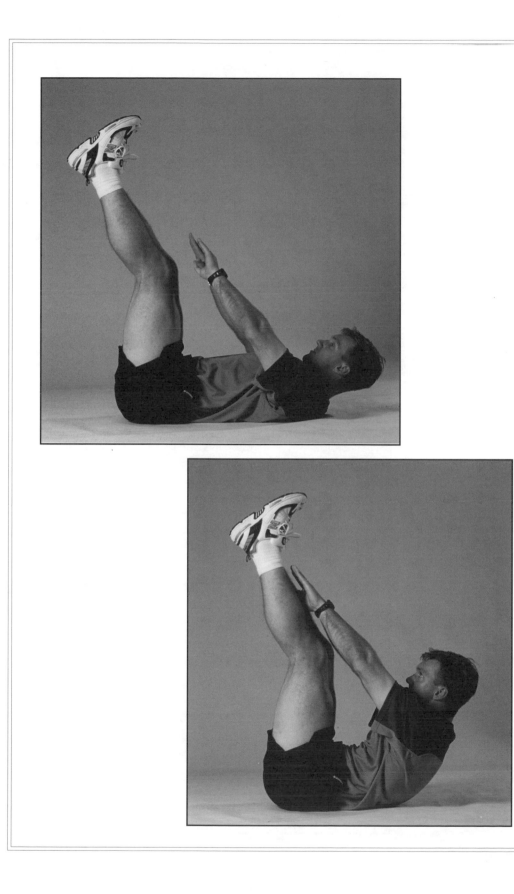

Advanced Crunch (Legs up)

Lie on your back with your legs straight in the air. Flex your stomach as you reach your hands to your toes. Avoid this exercise if you have had a previous lower back injury.

Advanced Right Elbow to Left Knee (Leg Up)

Crossing your left leg over your right leg, lift your right leg straight into the air. Bring your right elbow to your left knee by flexing your stomach and twisting to the left. Avoid this exercise if you have had a previous lower back injury.

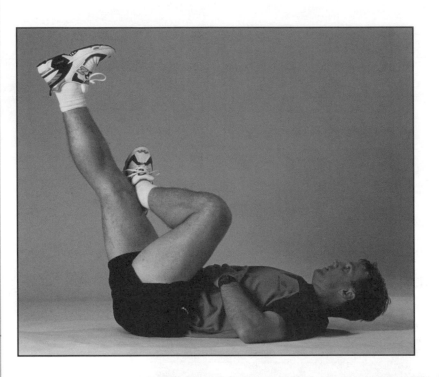

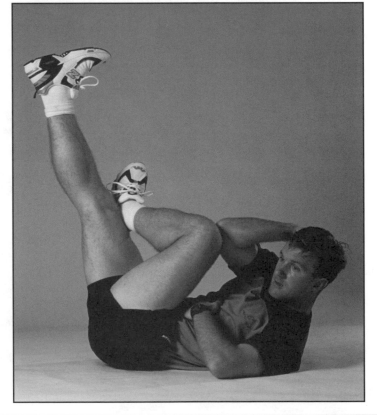

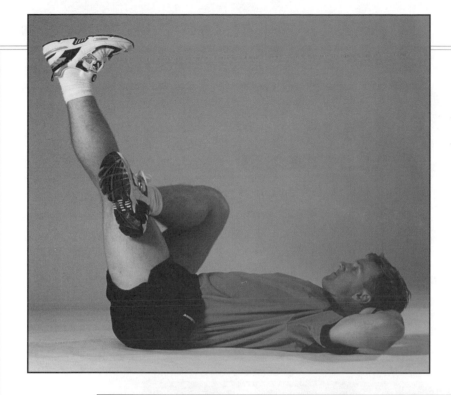

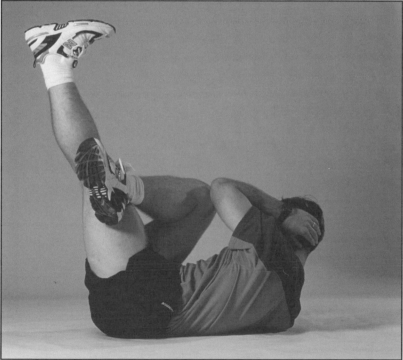

Advanced Left Elbow to Right Knee (Leg Up)

Crossing your right leg over your left leg, lift your left leg straight into the air. Bring your left elbow to your right knee by flexing your stomach and twisting to the right. Avoid this exercise if you have had a previous lower back injury.

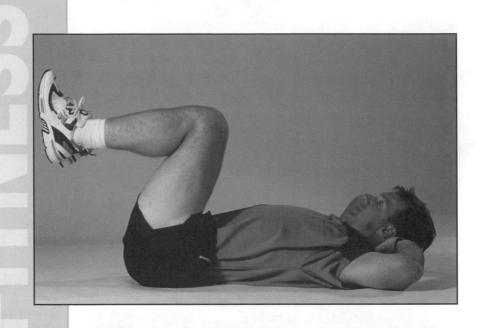

Advanced
Reverse (Legs Up)

Lie on your back and lift your butt and legs straight into the air. Reach your feet toward the ceiling as you flex your lower abdominal region. Avoid this exercise if you have had a previous lower back injury.

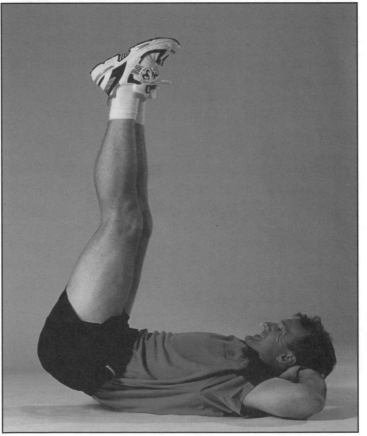

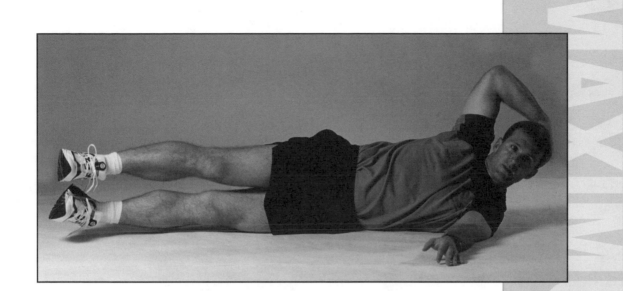

Side Oblique

Lie on your right side. Lift your legs and shoulders about three inches off the ground and hold them there. Switch sides to work the other love handle.

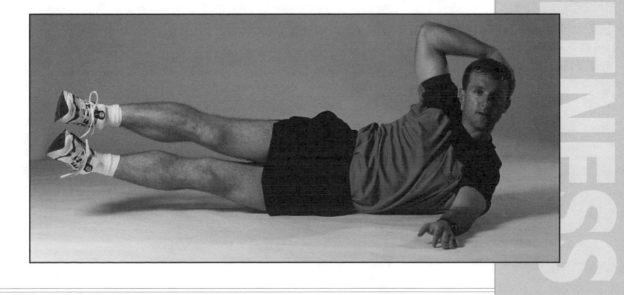

Inner-Outer Thigh Side Oblique

Add another muscle group to this love handle exercise by lifting your top leg and bottom shoulder to isolate the outer thigh. Bring your top leg forward and lift your bottom leg six to twelve inches as your raise your bottom shoulder to exercise both the obliques and inner and outer thighs.

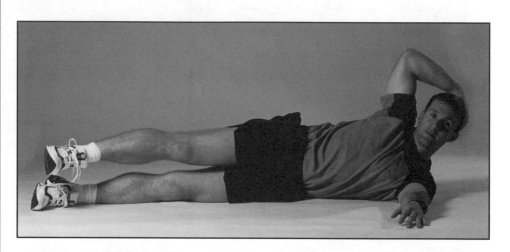

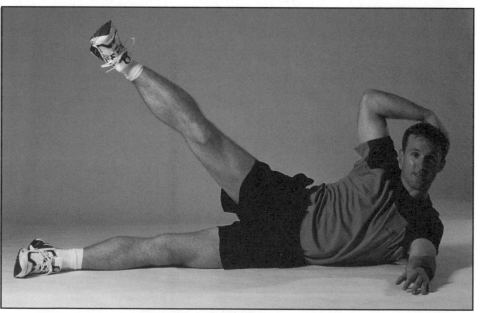

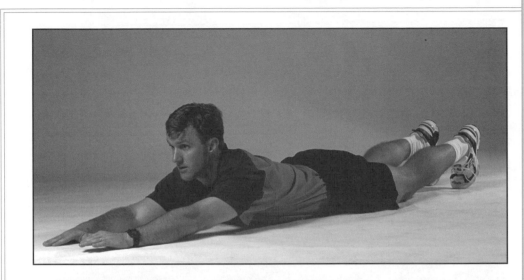

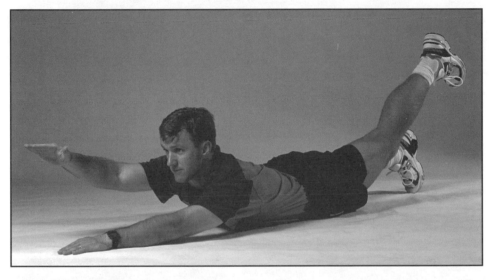

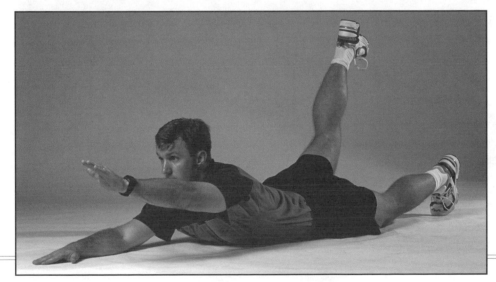

Prone Lower Back Exercise

Lie on your stomach with your arms extended over your head. Lift your right arm and your left leg off the ground at the same time. Switch arms/legs and repeat.

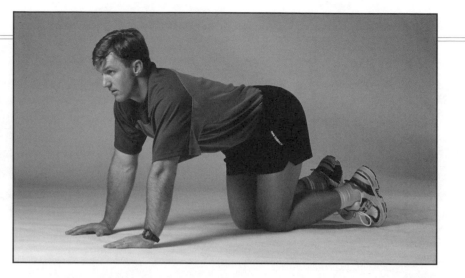

FITNESS

MAXIMUS

Prone Lower
Back Exercise # 2

On your hands and knees, lift your right arm and your left leg off the ground and extend them. Switch arms/legs and repeat.

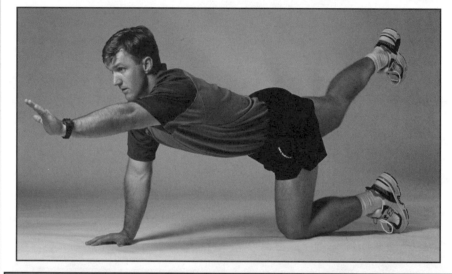

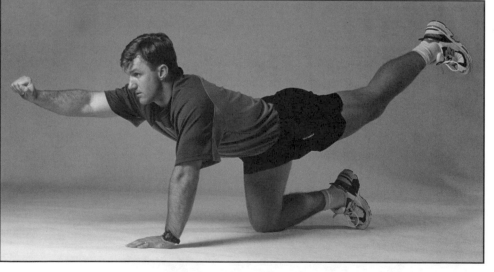

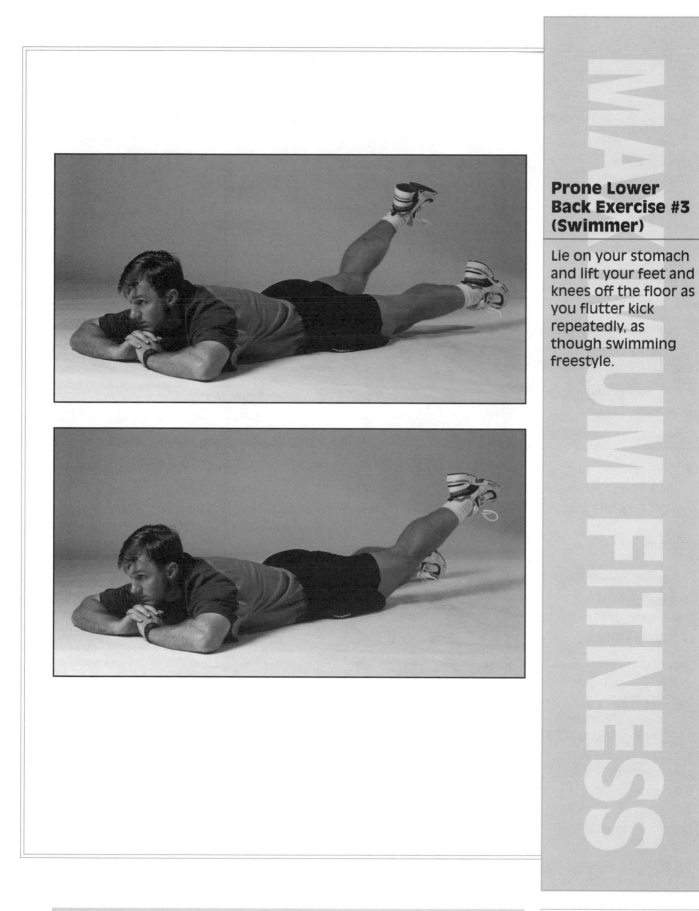

Prone Lower Back Exercise #3 (Swimmer)

Lie on your stomach and lift your feet and knees off the floor as you flutter kick repeatedly, as though swimming freestyle.

MAXIMUM FITNESS

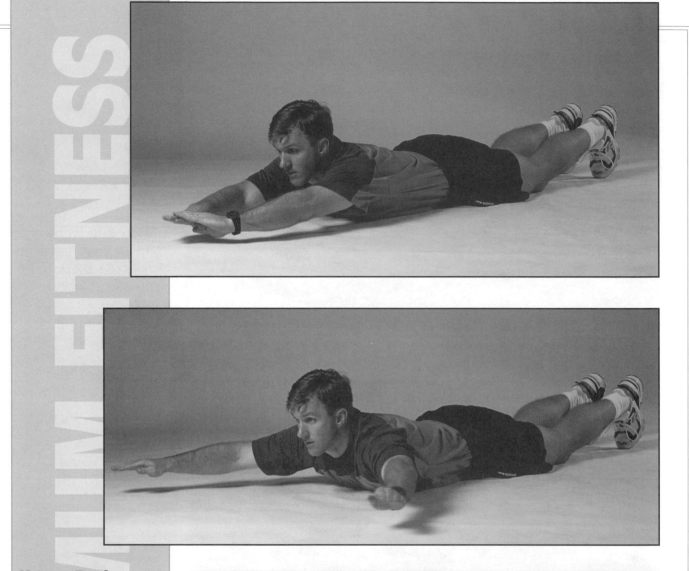

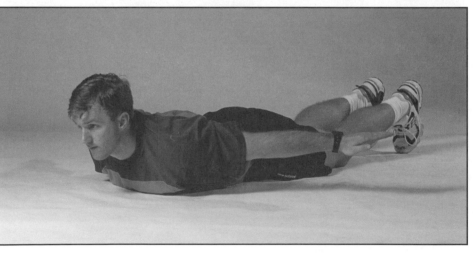

Upper Back Exercise #1 (Arm Haulers)

Lie on your stomach with your feet on the floor. Lift your chest slightly off the floor as you rotate your arms from your sides over your head for 30 seconds.

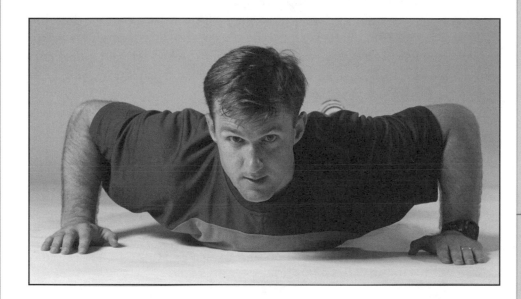

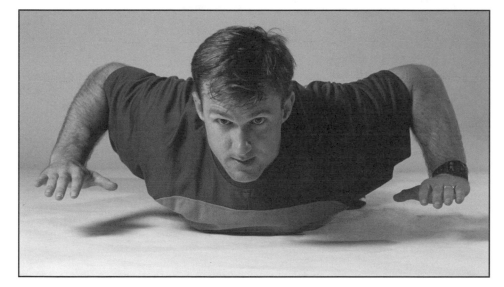

Upper Back Exercise #2 (Reverse Push-ups)

Lie on your stomach in the resting push-up position. Lift your hands off the floor instead of pushing down into the floor. This will strengthen the upper back muscles that oppose the chest muscles— rear deltoids and rhomboids.

MAXIMUM FITNESS

These exercises are potentially harmful to weak lower back muscles. Do not perform any of the following exercises if you are a beginner or have had ANY lower back injuries. These exercises are featured in this book because many readers are training to become Navy SEALs, Marines, Air Force PJ/ CCT's or Rangers. Such units perform these exercises several times a week in conjunction with heavy backpack runs. Strong lower back and abdominal muscles are essential for these units of the military. Only an advanced athlete should perform these exercises.

Tips to reduce strain on the lower back:

1. Lift your butt approximately one inch off the ground and place your hands underneath your butt bone.
2. Place your hands one on top of the other to lift the butt higher, therefore removing strain from the lower back.
3. Keep your knees straight and perform these exercises with the full range of motion of your hips. Your legs should range six inches from the floor to the vertical position.

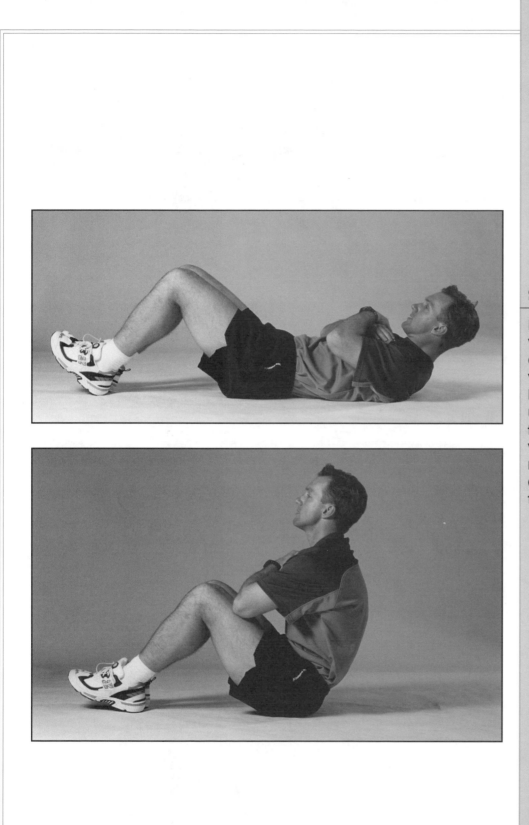

Situps

Lie on your back with your arms crossed over your chest, and your knees slightly bent. Raise your upper body off the floor by contracting your abdominal muscles. Touch your elbows to your thighs and repeat.

MAXI

Cross Situps

Lie on your back with your knees bent and your feet flat on the floor. With your hands behind your head or crossed over your chest, raise your upper body and twist your torso to touch your left elbow to your right knee. Return to the resting position and repeat, touching your right elbow to your left knee.

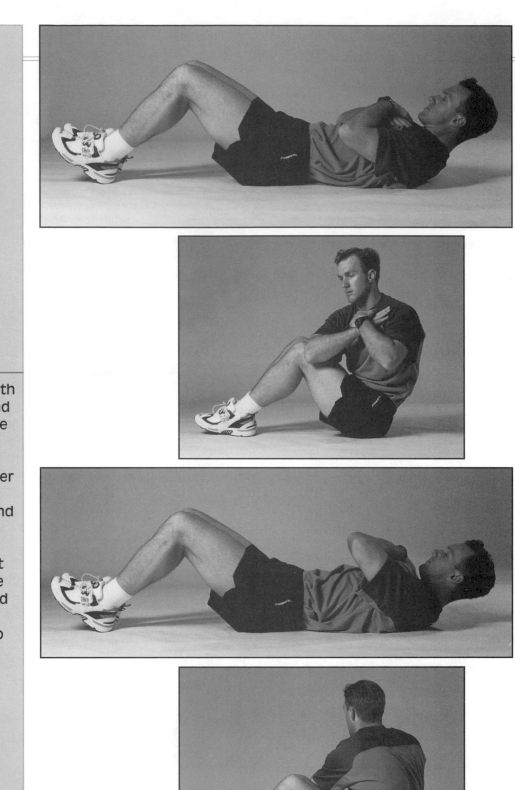

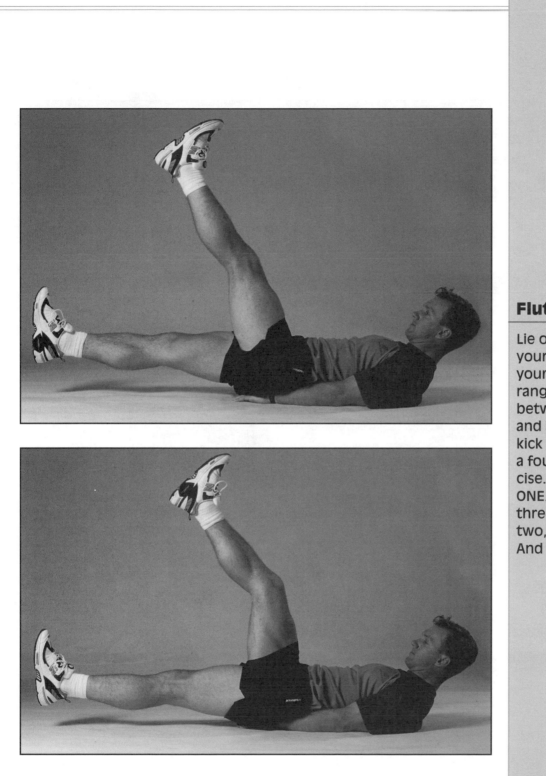

Flutter Kicks

Lie on your back with your hands under your hips. Keep your range of motion between six inches and 36 inches as you kick your legs. This is a four-count exercise. One, two, three, ONE. One, two, three, TWO. One, two, three, THREE. And so on.

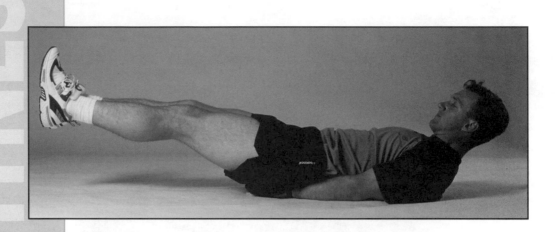

Leg Levers

Lie on your back and lift your feet six inches off the floor. Raise both legs approximately 36 inches off the ground, keeping your legs straight until your repetitions are complete.

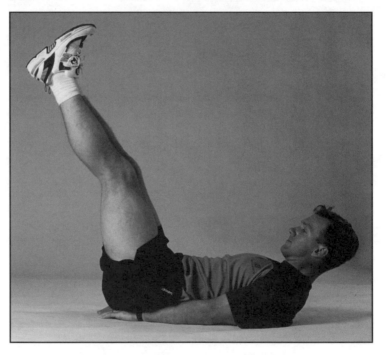

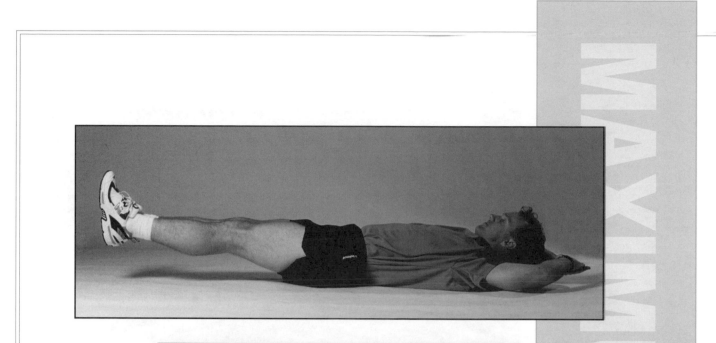

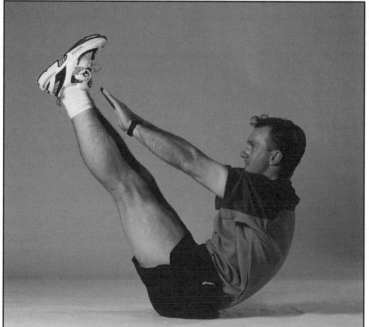

V-ups

Lie on your back with your legs straight. Bring your shoulders and legs as high as you can, reaching your hands toward your feet and back down to the ground.

Atomic Situps

Lie on your back and lift your feet six inches off the floor, in the same position as the leg lever. Pull your knees toward your chest while simultaneously lifting your upper body off the floor. This exercise is a combination of the situp and the leg lever.

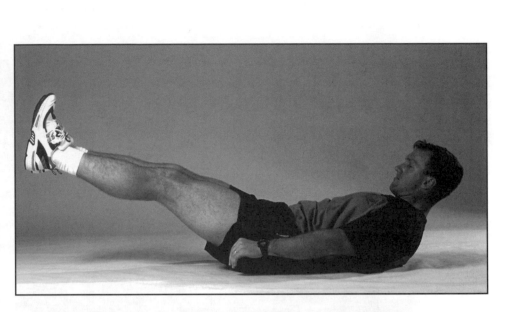

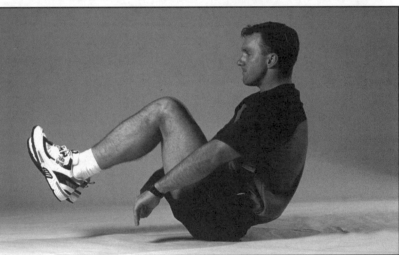

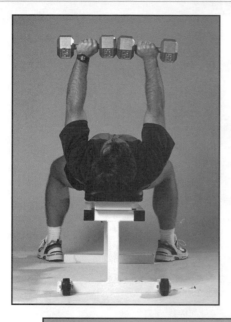

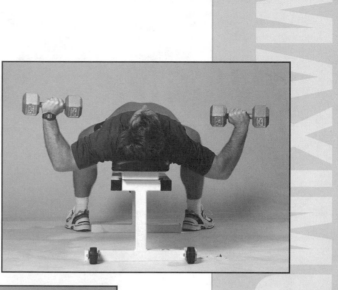

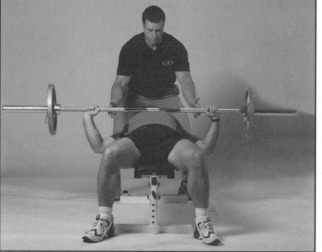

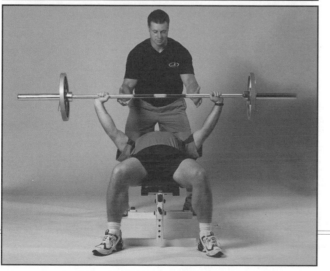

Flat Bench Press

Lying flat on the bench with your feet on the floor, grab either dumbbells or a barbell and lower it to your chest. Push the weight back up to starting position and repeat. Keep your arms approximately shoulder width apart to work your muscles with even distribution. Widen your grip to focus on your chest muscles and close your grip to focus on the triceps.

MAXIMUM

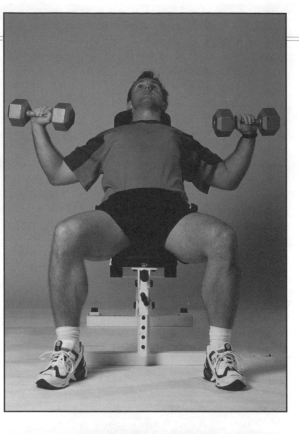

Dumbbell Bench/ Incline Flies

Using either the incline or flat bench, dumbbell flies are an excellent addition to your chest workout. Lie back holding a dumbbell in each hand. Bring the weights down and out to your sides. You will feel the stretch across your chest. Push back to starting position and repeat.

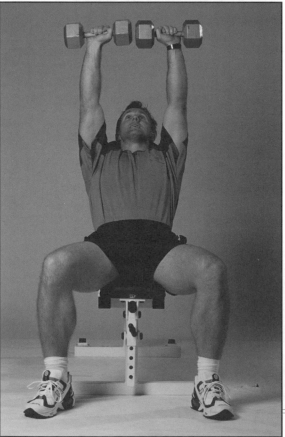

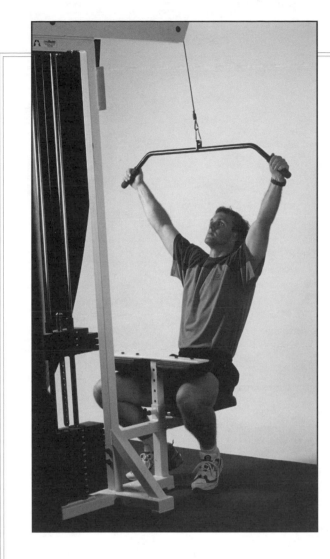

Pulldowns

Sit underneath the hanging bar of the pulldown machine. Use wide, shoulder width or close grips and pull the weighted bar down to your chest. Lean back slightly, pull your shoulders back, and push your chest forward to isolate the upper back muscles.

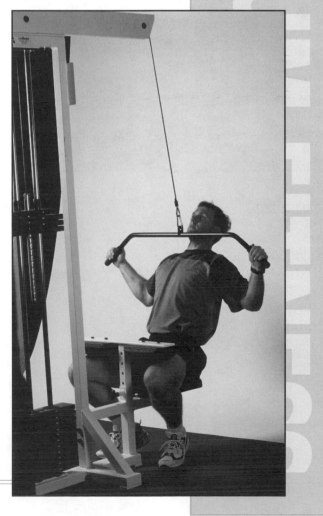

Pushdowns

Stand in front of the hanging weight. Push the weight from shoulder-height to waist-height, keeping your elbows tight by your sides.

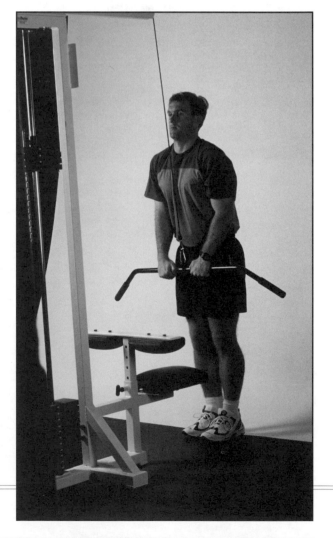

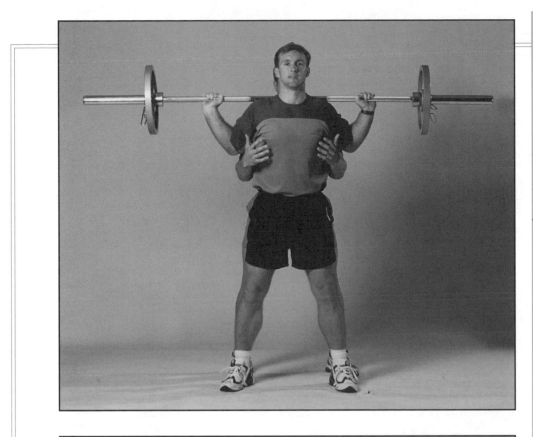

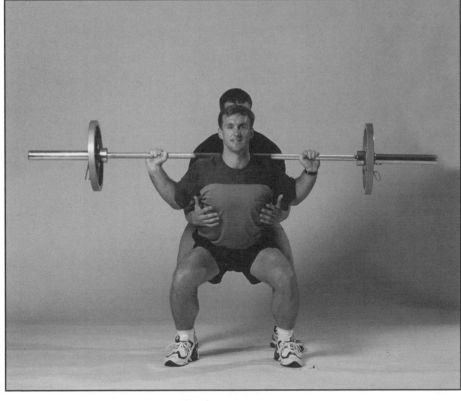

Squats

You can perform squats one of three ways: 1) without weight as described in the PT chapter, 2) using dumbbells, or 3) with a barbell across your back. Place the barbell perfectly balanced just below your shoulders (not on your neck). Look up at the ceiling, keeping your back straight and your knees bent. As you lower your body, be sure your knees remain over your feet and your buttocks extend behind you as though you were sitting on a chair.

MAXIMUM FITNESS

Leg Extensions

Sit down and place the leg machine cushions over your ankles. Lift as you slowly straighten your legs. Hold for one second and return the weight to the starting position.

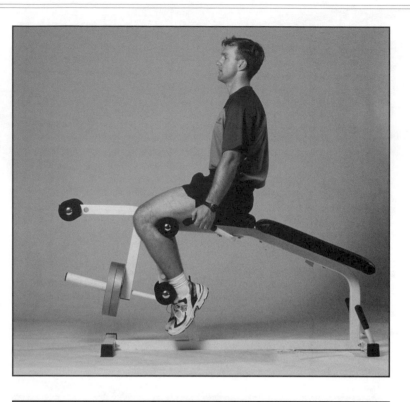

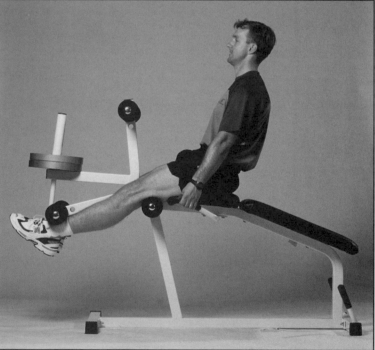

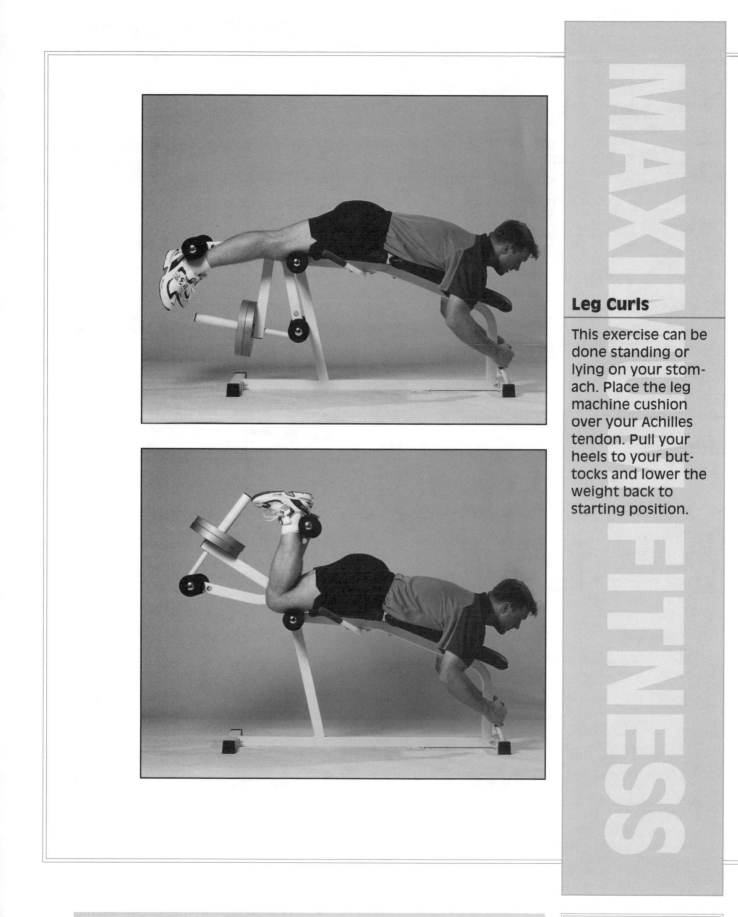

Leg Curls

This exercise can be done standing or lying on your stomach. Place the leg machine cushion over your Achilles tendon. Pull your heels to your buttocks and lower the weight back to starting position.

MAXIMUM

FITNESS

Reverse Fly

Lean forward at the waist while keeping your back flat. Be sure to keep your abdominal muscles tight. Start with the weights down in front of you. Concentrate on squeezing your shoulder blades together as you raise the weights out to the sides with your arms parallel to the ground. Muscles used: rear deltoids (shoulders).

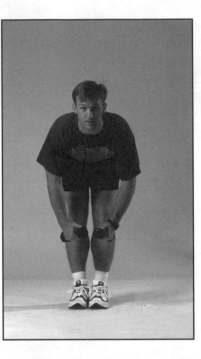
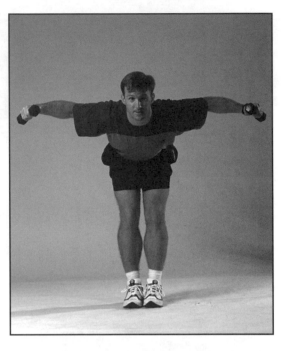
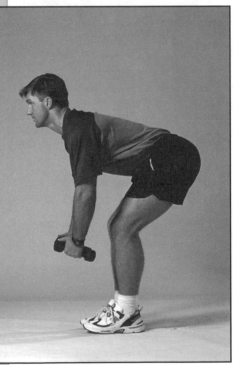
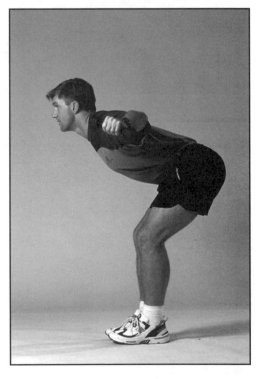

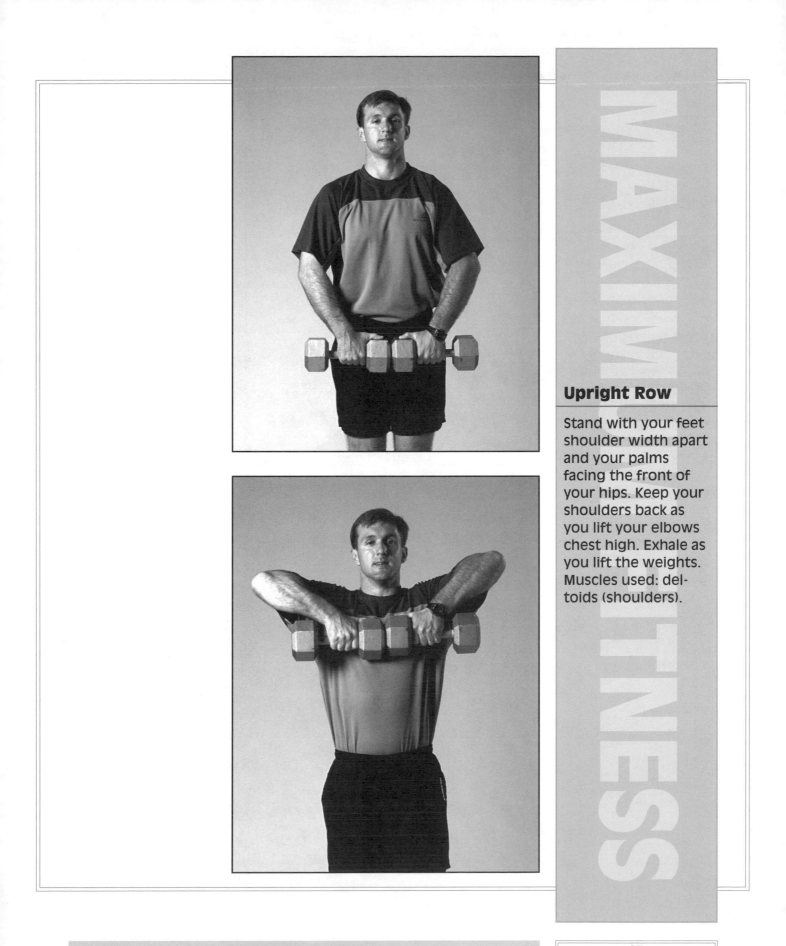

Upright Row

Stand with your feet shoulder width apart and your palms facing the front of your hips. Keep your shoulders back as you lift your elbows chest high. Exhale as you lift the weights. Muscles used: deltoids (shoulders).

Shoulder Shrug

Hold the weights by your sides. Keep your head up and eyes forward. Use a full range of motion as you lift your shoulders to your ears. This exercise helps develop and maintain good posture.

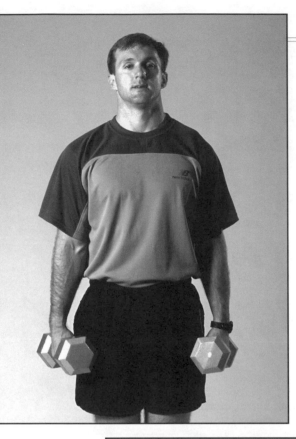

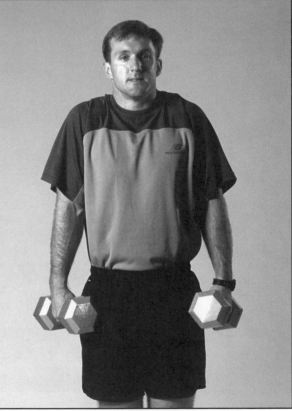

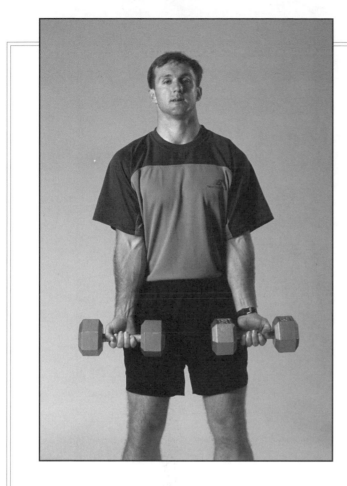

Biceps Curl

Hold dumbbells or a barbell with your palms facing upward. Use a complete range of motion as you lift the weights to your shoulders. Do not swing the weights. Isolate the movement in your elbows. Muscles used: biceps (arms).

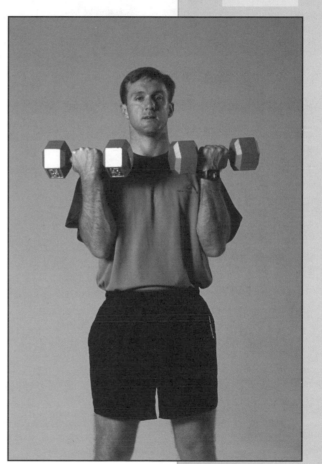

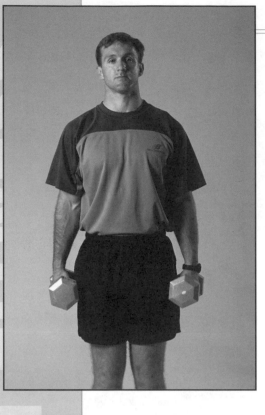

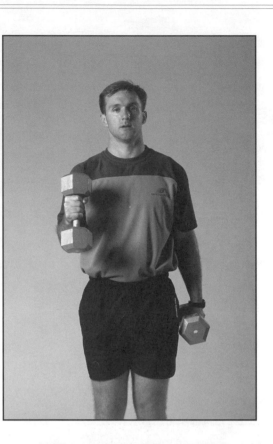

Hammer Curl

Begin this exercise in the same position as the biceps curl, except with your palms facing your hips. Alternate lifting each dumbbell as though you were running—"hip to lip." Use a complete range of motion and be careful not to swing the weights.

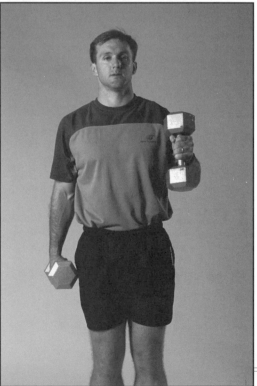

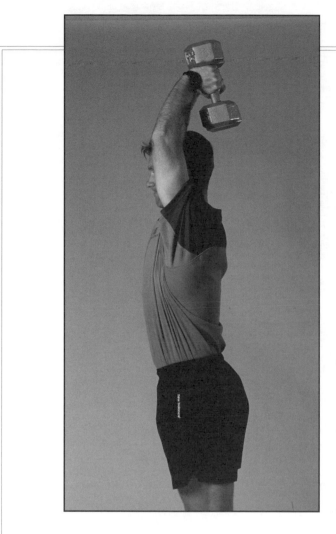

Hold a weight with both hands as you bring your arms over your head. Slowly lower the weight toward the back of your neck. Be sure your elbows remain pointed pointed toward the sky. Muscles used: triceps (back of the arm).

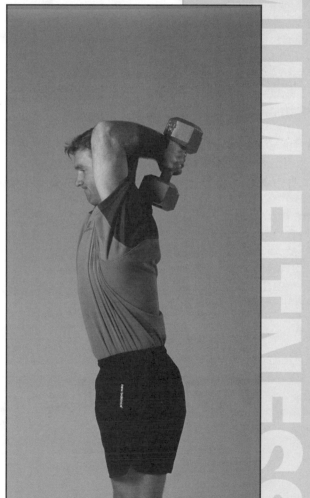

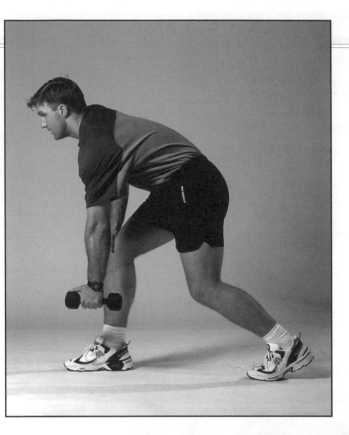

Bent-Over Row

With your right leg slightly in front of your left, bend forward at the waist and let your arms hang fully-extended. Holding a dumbbell in your left hand, pull the weight up to waist-height. Keep your trunk stable throughout the full range of motion. Repeat on opposite side. Muscles used: latissimus dorsi (back) and biceps (arms).

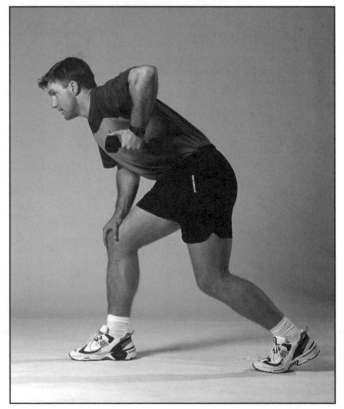

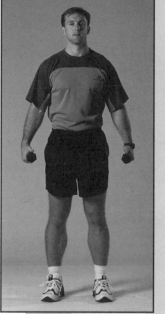

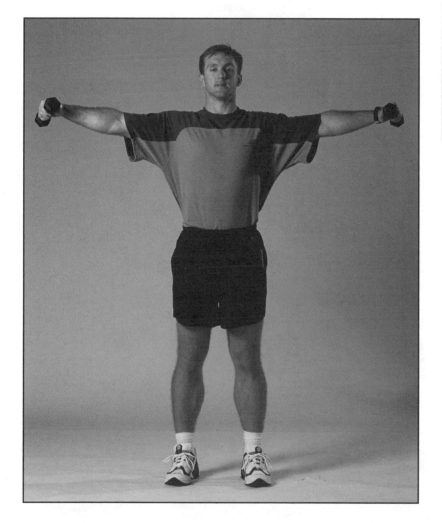

Lateral Raise

This safe and effective shoulder exercise requires light weights—five pound dumbbells maximum. Keep your knees slightly bent, shoulder back, and chest high. Lift the weights out to your sides parallel to the ground in a smooth, controlled motion, keeping your palms facing down. Repeat ten times. Continue with the remaining shoulder exercises without taking a rest.

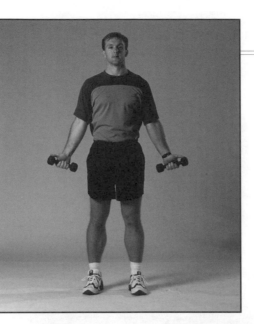

Thumbs Up

After completing the regular lateral raises, perform ten lateral raises with your thumbs up. With your palms facing away from you, extend the weights from your hips to shoulder-height.

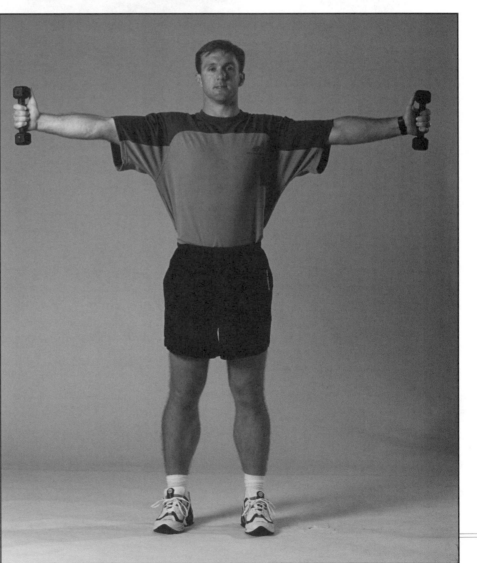

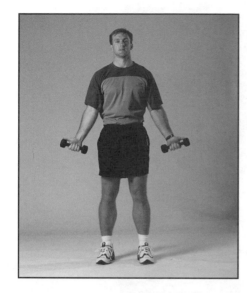

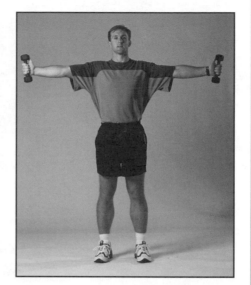

Continue the workout with side lateral raises. As you lift your arms up, keep your thumbs pointing upward. Once your arms are shoulder-height, turn your thumbs pointing down as you lower the weights. Repeat ten times, as you lead the direction with your thumbs.

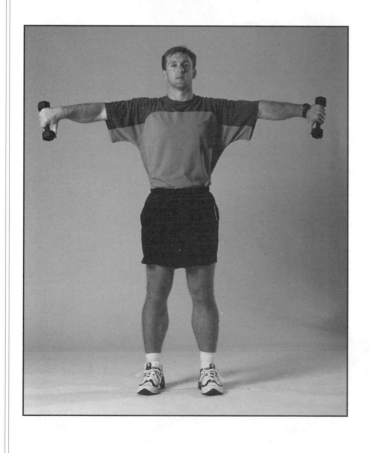

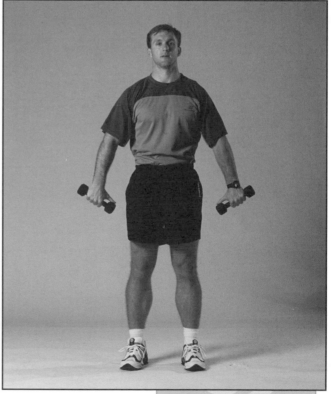

Front Raise (Thumbs Up)

Lift the dumbbells from your waist to shoulder-height with your arms out in front of you, keeping your thumbs facing upward. Repeat ten times. Muscles used: front deltoids.

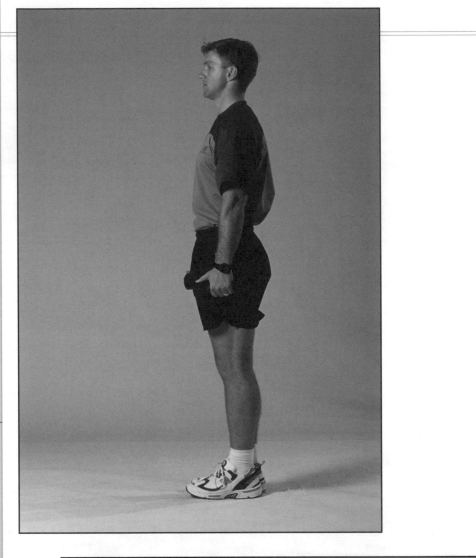

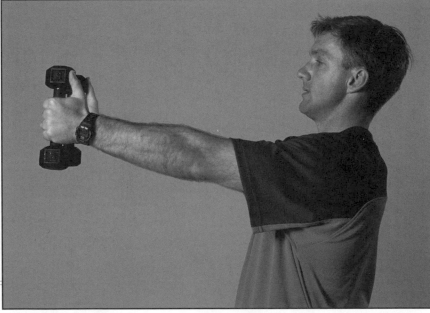

MAXIMUM

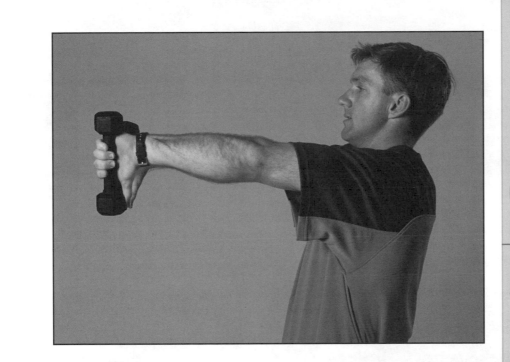

Front Raise (Thumbs Up / Down)

Perform the thumbs up/down exercise with your arms out in front of you. Repeat ten times.

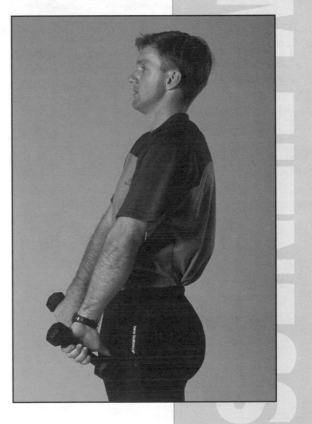

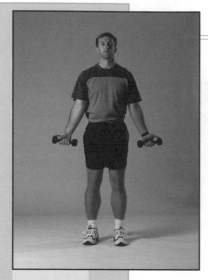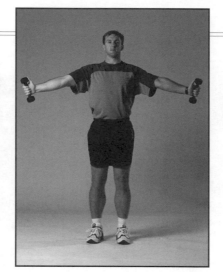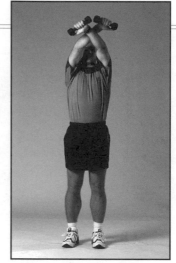

Cross Overs

Stand with your arms relaxed at your sides and your palms facing up. Bring your arms over your head as though you were doing a jumping jack. Cross your arms in front of your head and return to the starting position. Repeat ten times.

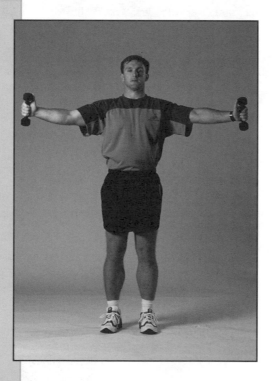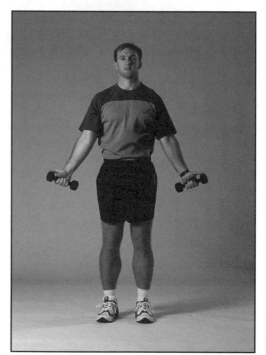

MAXIMUM

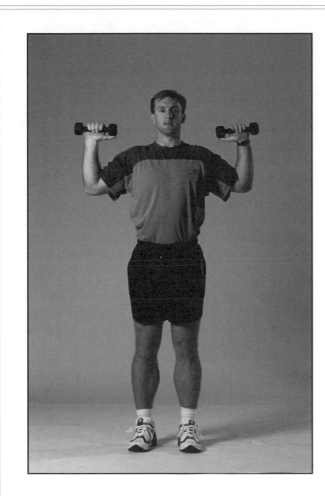

Military Press

Stand shoulder width apart with your knees slightly bent to reduce the strain on your lower back. Exhale as you push the weights over your head. Slowly lower your arms to shoulder-height and repeat ten final repetitions. Muscles used: deltoids (shoulders) and triceps (back of arm).

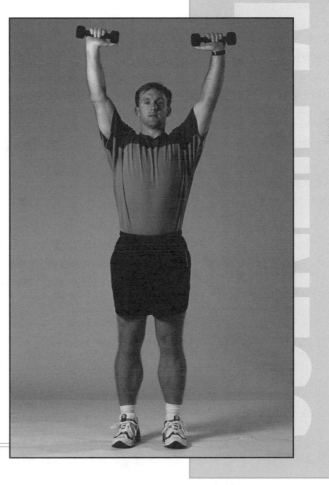

PT Workout Plans

Maximum Fitness—The Complete Guide to Cross Training contains over 70 different workouts with over 90 different exercises. Understandably, the magnitude of these workouts can be somewhat overwhelming. Therefore, this chapter is dedicated to explaining the various calisthenics workouts and exercises featured in this book.

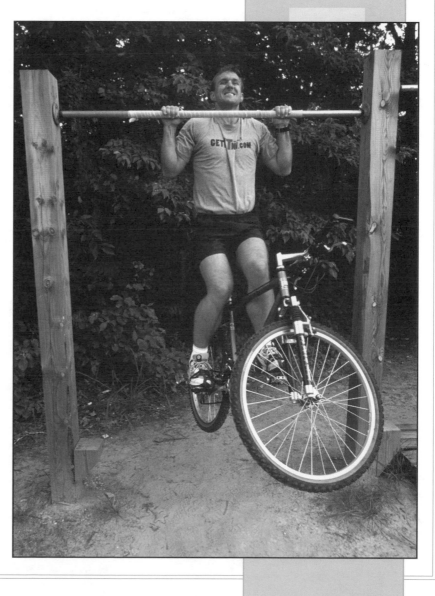

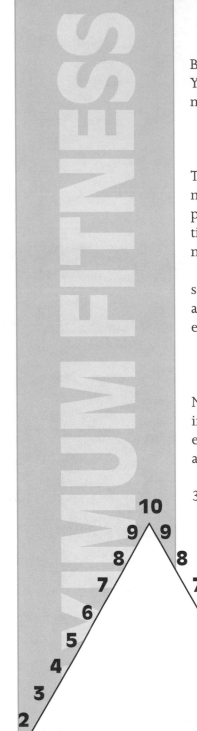

MAXIMUM FITNESS

Rest Day / Stretch

Built into the workout schedules are days to relax and stretch tight muscles. You should exercise FIVE to SIX days and rest ONE to TWO days per week. You may choose which days to rest or follow the suggested program.

Sets x Reps Concept

Throughout the workouts, you will notice the phrase "sets x reps." This common fitness term abbreviates the phrase "sets of repetitions," meaning you perform a specified number of squats, for example, a specified number of times. On Week #1 of the calisthenics workout, you will do 3 x 20 of squats, meaning you will perform 20 squat repetitions a total of three times.

Whenever you see "sets x reps" in these workouts, give yourself a 30 to 60 second rest between sets. If there are several exercises within a workout that all contain the same number of sets to complete, you may alternate between exercises with little rest.

The PT Pyramid Workouts

Notice the numbering of the PT pyramid— ascending up one side, descending down the other. Each number represents a step in the pyramid. Consider each step a "set" of your workout. The goal is to climb the pyramid to the top, and then all the way back down.

The bottom of the pyramid contains "pull-ups x 1, push-ups x 2, situps x 3." This means that at each "set" or step of the pyramid, you perform one pull-up for every step you are on, 2 push-ups, and 3 situps.

Start at the bottom left of the pyramid, at number one. For this set, perform 1 pull-up / 2 push-ups / 3 situps. Then, move to the step number two and perform 2 pull-ups / 4 push-ups / 6 situps. At step three, perform 3 pull-ups / 6 push-ups / 9 situps. For each set, multiple the set number by one for the number of pull-ups, by two for number of push-ups, and by three for the number of situps. Keep progressing until you reach the top of the pyramid, or your MAX. At step number ten, you perform 10 pull-ups / 20 push-ups / 30 situps. Now, begin working your way back down the other side of the pyramid from step number nine. Keep going until you have reach number one again.

Pull-ups x 1, Push-ups x 2, Situps x 3

The Pull-up Pyramid

Follow the PT pyramid routine, resting between pull-up sets for no longer than one minute. Continue the pull-ups until you have reached your maximum, then resort to negative pull-ups for the remainder of the workout. Instead of resting between sets, try to do at least 25 abdominal exercises during your rest periods.

50-Pull-up Workout

 The objective of the 50- and 100-pull-up workout is to perform as many pull-ups in as few sets as possible. Set your own goals, but aim for two to three sets during the 50-pull-up workout and six to eight sets for the 100-pull-up workout. For certain weeks, you may have to repeat 50 pull-ups. Use the break between sets to do abdominal or cardiovascular exercises. This workout can also be done with assisted pull-ups.

Mega-MAX Workout

This workout can be done with pull-ups alone or integrating push-ups, dips, and situps. Begin by performing the maximum number of pull-ups, push-ups and dips that you can do. Then, without rest, start the second set of MAX pull-ups, subtracting two repetitions from your original maximum effort (MAX -2); MAX push-ups minus ten (MAX - 10); and MAX dips minus four (MAX - 4). Set three will further decrease the maximum repetitions of each exercise. Continue this workout until you can no longer perform any pull-ups, push-ups, or dips.

MAXIMUM FITNESS

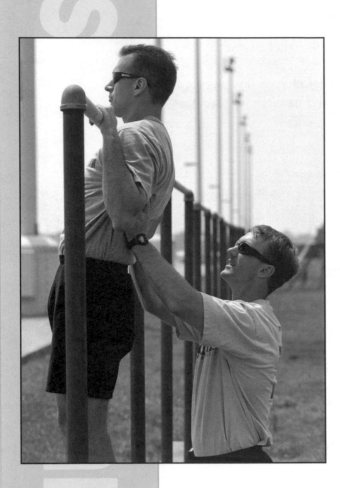

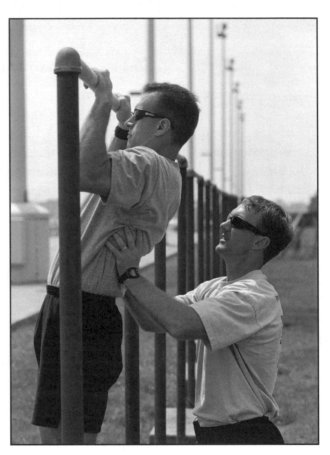

Proper Spotting Technique

This is one of two ways to spot your buddy during pullups. Lift your buddy over the bar and let him come down on his own to the count of "Five Mississippis, Four Mississippis, . . ."

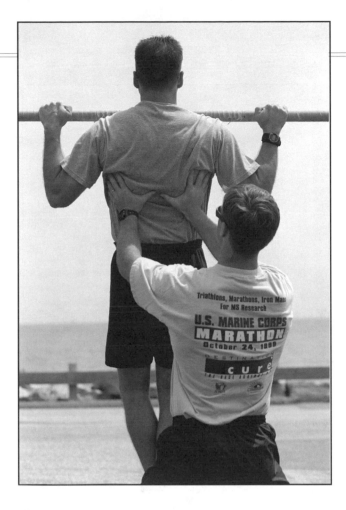

Negatives

Negative pull-ups should be done if you cannot do pull-ups. For the majority of men and women whom cannot do pull-ups, this workout will challenge you. This is the second step to doing pull-ups. After easily completing the required reps with assisted pull-ups, try a negative pull-up routine. A negative pull-up is half of a regular pull-up. Bring your chin over the bar, either by standing on a chair or having someone lift you. Once you are above the bar, resist gravity as you slowly lower yourself down for a count of five seconds. This conditions your arms to support your weight. Negative pull-ups can build up your strength to complete your first pull-up or to increase the number of regular pull-ups you can perform.

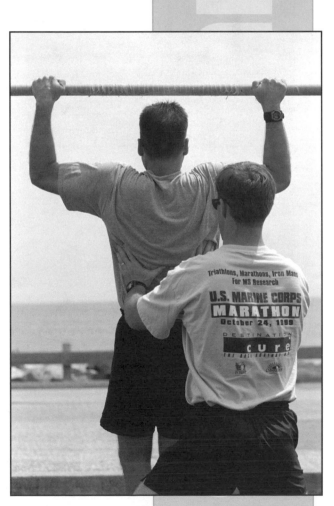

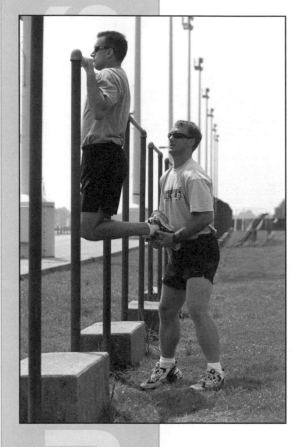

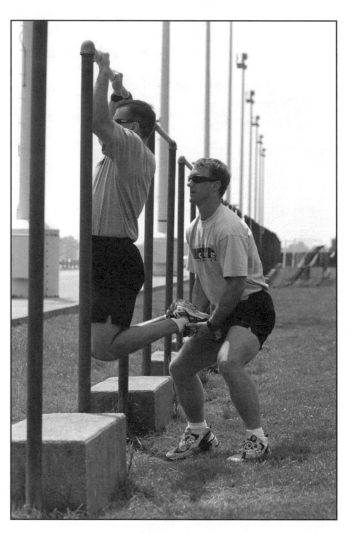

Grab Feet Spotting Technique

This is another way to spot your buddy. While he hangs under the bar, grab his feet. Allow your buddy to straighten his legs. This will help him lift over the bar.

Push-up/Crunch Superset

The superset is an excellent way to achieve extraordinary repetitions of push-ups and crunches! Each set of six exercises should be completed within a two-minute period. For example, the superset during Week # 3 of the calisthenics workout consists of:

Set #1:

5	regular push-ups
15	regular crunches
5	wide push-ups
15	reverse crunches
5	triceps push-ups
15	regular crunches

You should finish this two-minute superset with at least 30 to 45 seconds remaining. Use this time to stretch or drink some water. This circuit will be repeated five times for a total time of ten minutes. However, you will achieve 75 push-ups and 225 abdominal exercises in that time! Some of the superset workouts will increase in time and reps totaling over 600 push-ups and crunches in as little as 40 minutes.

REST

There is no rest time while on the two-minute clock. Do your set as quickly as possible, but watch your form. Do not jeopardize form for a faster superset time. This is a great time-saver workout if you are too busy to exercise for 30 to 45 minutes. Take 10 to 20 minutes and be amazed as you perform 100 to 200 push-ups and crunches in that time. If you finish your superset in one minute and 30 seconds, you get 30 seconds to rest before you begin the next set.

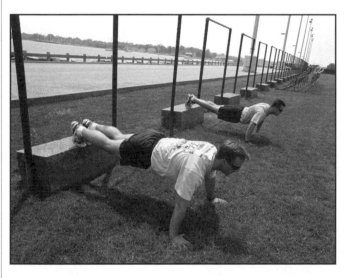

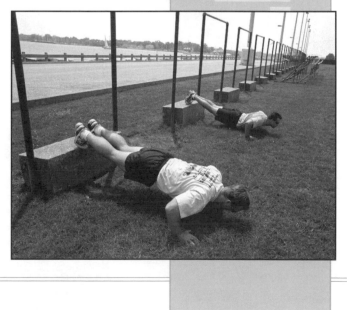

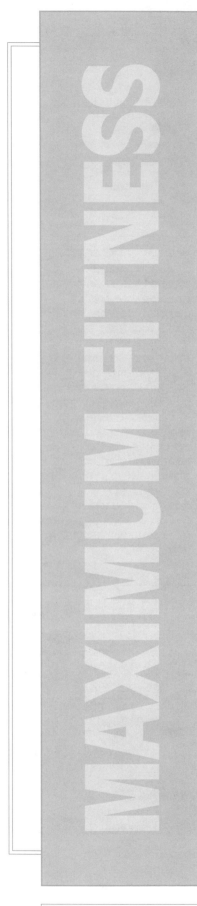

Lower Body PT

There are three main calisthenics exercises on lower body PT days—squats, lunges, and calf raises. Different variations of each of these exercises are mixed with running, biking, and swimming with fins. Use dumbbells to increase the difficulty of this workout in upcoming weeks.

These workouts can be accomplished two ways:

Alternating Sets

Perform the required reps of squats, lunges, and calf raises. After completing the first set, take a minute to rest before beginning the second set of each exercise. Repeat if required.

Regular Sets

Perform the required number of squat repetitions. Take a 30-second to one-minute rest, and then repeat the squats again until all sets are completed. Continue to perform lunges in the same fashion, then calf raises.

Another important element of leg PT is biking. Use either a stationary bike with varied manual resistance capability or a regular bicycle. Attachments are available at sporting good stores to convert a regular bike into a stationary bike for inside use.

Lifecycle Pyramid Workout

The first bike workout is the Lifecycle pyramid. This routine requires you adjust the tension of your bike every minute of your workout. I prefer the manual mode of the Lifecycle and start peddling at 80 to 90 RPMs (revolutions per minute). This workout starts off easy as you peddle at level one for one minute. For the second minute, increase to level two and continue to level twelve. Then, descend the pyramid with the same routine, repeating each level for one minute. This workout should only take 23 minutes to advance from level one to level twelve, then back to level one again.

Pushing and Pulling Bike Workout

This workout requires a bike with foot locks or straps on the pedals. These are necessary for your legs to pull the pedals, instead of just pushing them. This is an intense hamstring workout, so be sure you properly stretch before and after this routine. This workout takes approximately 20 to 30 minutes and requires you alternate pushing for one minute and pulling for one minute.

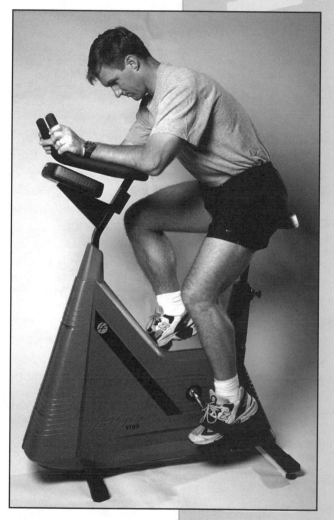

Bike/Leg PT/Abs MAX

This workout alternates biking, squats, lunges, and calf exercises. Bike for three to five minutes, then perform one minute of squats, one minute of lunges (30 seconds per leg), and one minute of calf exercises. You are periodically required to perform abdominal exercise or change the tension level on the bike. Repeat the cycle for the specified number of repetitions.

Be careful to stretch well before and after this workout—muscle pulls and tears are common if not properly stretched.

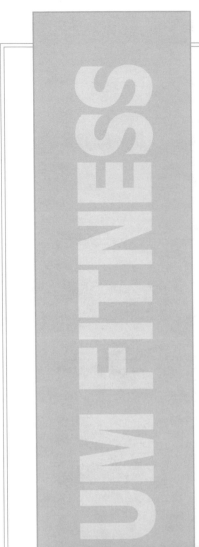

Swimming or Running and Leg PT

In the hardcore 13-week PT cycle, leg PT is mixed with a track workout. Sprinting, jogging (interval training), and resting are integrated with several variations of squats, lunges, and calf exercises. In the pool, the workout requires a 100-yard swim, followed by a series of squats, lunges, and calf exercises as well. Usually, swimming with fins will follow to further exhaust your legs.

Circuit Workouts

There are several different circuit routines in this workout program. A circuit routine is designed to advance as quickly as possible through a workout. There are no rest periods in a circuit workout until the end. Your muscles will have time to rest as you rotate exercises, rarely using the same muscle groups twice in a row. In this book, there are full-body PT circuits, upper body PT circuits, and weights mixed with PT circuits. These circuits are the fastest, yet most intense workouts in the book. Generally, in as little as 12 to 18 minutes, you will reach complete muscle failure.

PT With The Clock

This type of workout is designed to help students ace a physical fitness test of pull-ups, push-ups, and situps. By performing as many reps as you can of each exercise in a certain time limit, you will learn the pace required to achieve 100 push-ups and 100 situps in two minutes. By using the clock as your training guide, you will become accustomed to doing maximum reps in a time period, which will further increase your scores as you continue to practice this type of training.

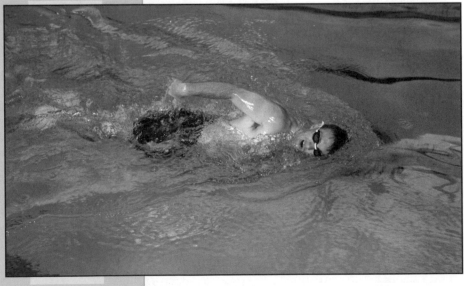

Swimming, Running, and Biking Workout Plans

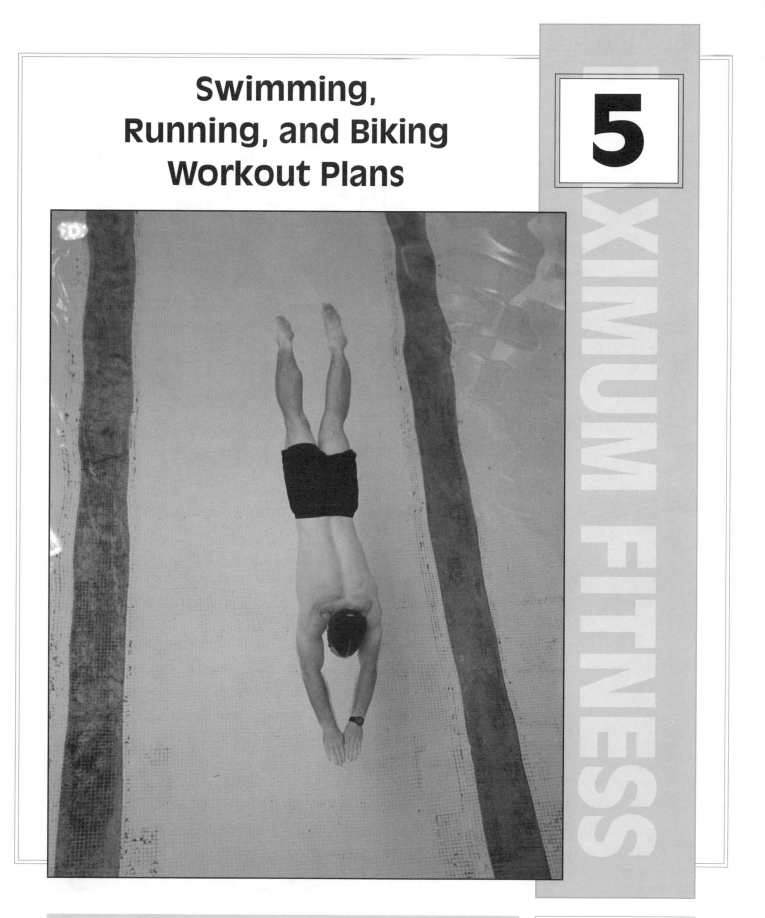

MAXIMUM FITNESS

Hypoxic pyramids (strokes / breath) are probably the most challenging cardiovascular workout in the 52-week workout. This workout not only makes ordinary swimming seem easy, it make your swimming, running, and overall endurance stronger. By limiting your breathing, you mimic training at high altitudes. Therefore, when you test breathing regularly, your body will react similar to a high-altitude athlete returning to sea level to compete. My resting heart rate drops significantly (38 to 50 bpm) when I perform this type of training regularly.

This workout increases in difficulty after each 100 meters you swim. By adding two strokes per breath every 100 meters, the need to breathe will become significantly more demanding. Climb the pyramid using each set of 100 meters as a step. For each step, add two more strokes per breath. You breathe less as you ascend each step of the pyramid until you reach the maximum of ten strokes per breath. Each arm pull is a stroke, therefore, a step with four strokes per breath would count: one, two, three, four, breathe—translating to left arm pull, right, left, right, breathe.

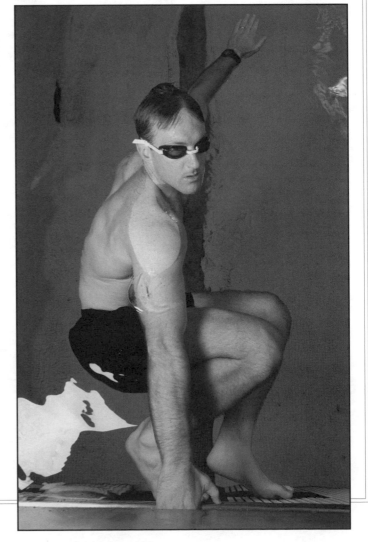

10

8   8

6   6

4   4

2   2

(strokes per breath)
100m or 200m

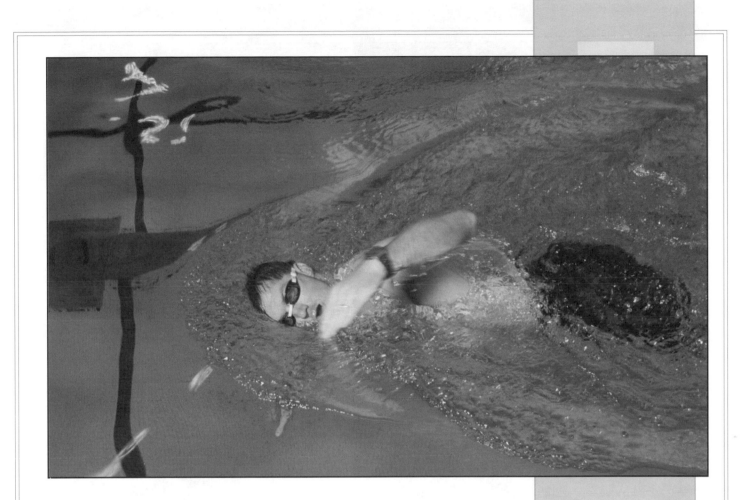

I have found that holding my breath for at least half the stroke count before slowly exhaling can significantly reduce the difficulty of completing the pyramid. It will take time before you can perform this workout with no rest at all. When you begin this workout, take a 20- to 30-second rest between steps if necessary.

The **strokes per length hypoxic workout** requires swimming a designated distance with a specific number of breaths. For instance, you'll swim 50 meters breathing only four times, then three times, then two, then only once, for a total of 200 meters. Repeat this workout several more times to complete 1000 meters.

Over / under (25 yards) is a term describing the method used to swim from one end of the pool to the other. "Over" means swimming on top of the water either using the freestyle or sidestroke. "Under" means swimming either underwater or freestyle without taking breaths. This workout is extremely challenging and potentially dangerous. *Do not perform this workout alone. In fact, never swim underwater alone or without a lifeguard. It is easy to blackout while exerting yourself without regular breaths.*

Swim PT is a great way to combine swimming and upper body PT into the same workout. Swim the specified distances (usually 100 yards or meters), get out of the pool, and perform push-ups, abdominal exercises, and pull-outs. Repeat this sequence a minimum of ten times.

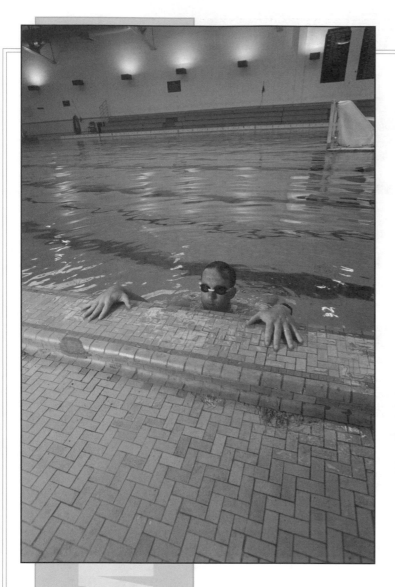

To perform a **pullout**, grab the edge of the pool with both hands, and lift your upper body out of the water until your hips are touching the pool's edge.

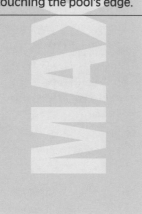

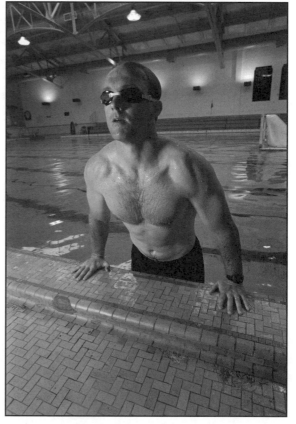

Swimming with fins is the best leg workout available to tone and strengthen your hamstrings, hip flexors, and ankles in only a few months. Swim the regular sidestroke with the following differences:

Constant flutter kicks

With fins on your feet, your biggest source of power will naturally be your legs, so kick constantly to propel through the water.

Open water swimming in a straight line

Approximately every five strokes, look forward to be sure you are swimming in a straight line. This is not necessary in a swimming pool; however, it is important when surface swimming in the open ocean to have a visual reference for accuracy.

Sample workout

Swim 500 yards with fins, then 500 yards without fins using the stroke of your choice.

MAXIMUM FITNESS

FITNESS

The term "sprints" in swimming, means swimming at maximum speed a designated distance for a specified number of repetitions. Try to limit your rest periods to 20 to 30 seconds. For instance, "200m x 3" means swim a 200-meter sprint, rest for 20 to 30 seconds, and repeat the sprint twice more for a total of three times. The preferred stroke is freestyle, although you may choose any stroke you like. Swim sprints with leg and upper body PT can be incorporated into a hardcore swim/PT workout. If you mix leg PT with swimming, focus on flutter kicks and breaststroke kicks to target the legs.

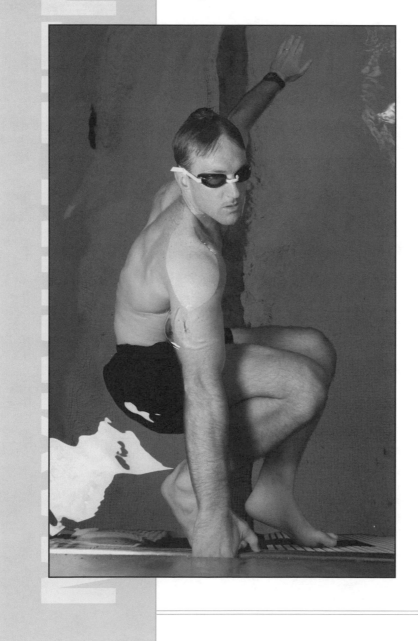

Run/Swim/Run

As one of the best endurance training workouts, this triathlon combines only running and swimming, although biking may be substituted for running. Despite the simplicity of this workout, the second run is challenging, especially if you are swimming with fins. Try not to divide the workout into swimming in the morning and running in the afternoon; however, if necessary, you may break up the workout to fit your schedule. An example of one of most difficult run-swim-run workouts is:

1. Run four miles
2. Swim 3000 meters with fins
3. Run four miles

Run-Swim/PT-Run

A mix of two old favorites—swim PT and run/swim/run—this routine is one of the most demanding upper body and cardiovascular workouts in the 52-week program, especially with the optional hypoxic pyramid between each set of 100-meter swims.

1. Run three miles (18 to 24 minutes)
1. Repeat ten times
   a. Swim 100 meters
   b. Twenty abdominal exercises of your choice
   c. Twenty push-ups
   d. Five pullouts
3. Run three miles (20 to 24 minutes)

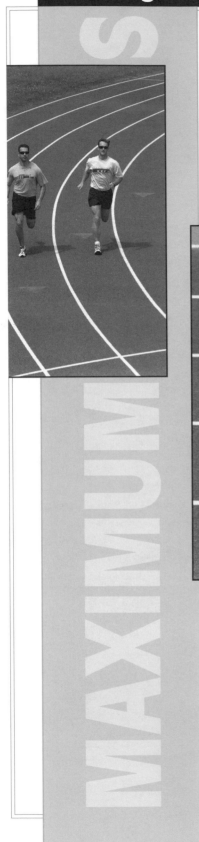

MAXIMUM

Three-Mile and Four-Mile Track Workouts

While a track is not needed, you need to measure your running distance to time your workout. The three- and the four-mile track workouts each begin with a one-mile jog. Following the warm-up jog, sprint a quarter-mile at maximum speed. Aim for a quarter-mile in 60 seconds.

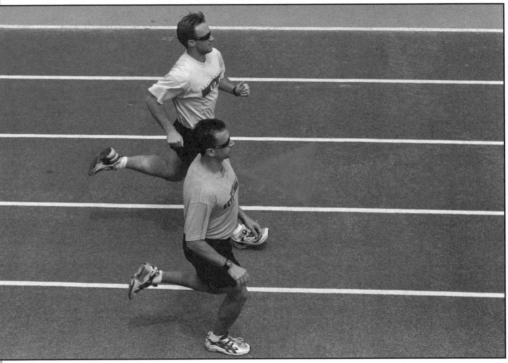

Then, jog another quarter-mile at the same pace as your warm-up mile (seven to eight minutes per mile). Repeat once more for the three-mile track workout and twice more for the four-mile track workout.

Finally, sprint one-eighth mile at maximum speed, followed by a one-eighth mile jog. Your goal is to decrease your running time for any distance. Repeat the one-eighth mile jog, and sprint three more times for the three-mile track workout and five more times for the four-mile track workout.

Running is probably the most dangerous exercise in this book because of its exertion on your body. Even athletes who run several miles a week are at risk. Fifty percent of avid runners will suffer injury this year. Most people do not know how to run properly. One of the best books I have read on running techniques and training is Alberto Salazar's **Treadmill Training and Workout Guide** (Hatherleigh Press, 2000). Here are a few tips to help you pick up the pace and avoid injury:

Breathing

Take deep inhalations and exhalations to supply your body with the oxygen it needs. People often breathe too shallow while running, causing hyperventilation. Slow down if necessary, but concentrate on your breathing. Deep inhales and full exhales are essential to release carbon dioxide from your lungs and slow your heart rate.

Stride and Heel / Toe Contact

Open your stride until you land on your heel and roll across your foot, pushing off the ground with your toes. Many people run flat-footed or on their toes, causing stress to their lower backs, hips, knees and ankles. This can be eliminated with a simple audio test: If you can hear your feet hitting the ground when you run, your foot position is incorrect. Your shoes should sound as though they are rolling on the ground.

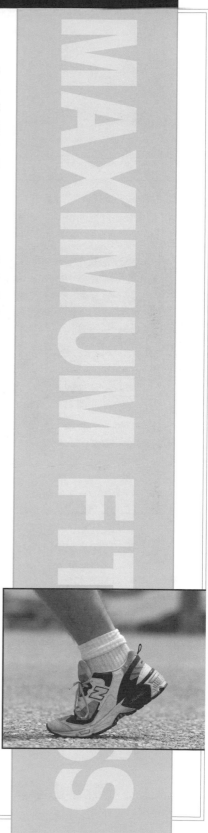

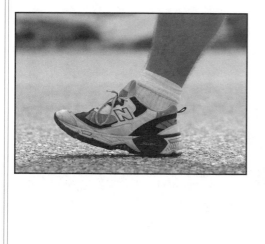

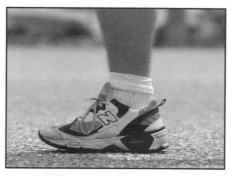

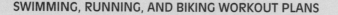

Arm Swing

You should have a relaxed, but pronounced arm swing. Swing your hands from chest-high to slightly past your hips. The term "hip to lip" is a good way to remember this range of motion while running. Keep your arms slightly bent but not flexed.

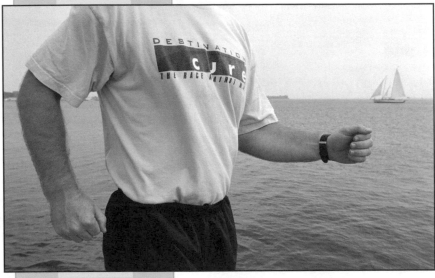

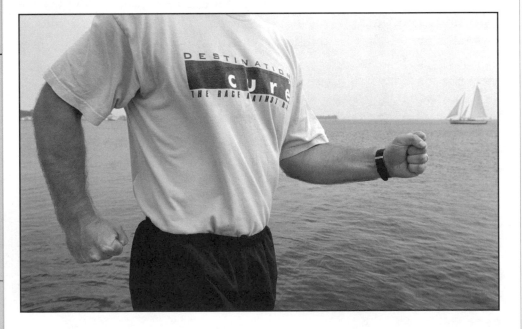

RELAXED UPPER BODY

Relax your fists, arms, shoulders, and face. Often, people clinch their fists and grit their teeth when they run causing oxygenated blood needed for your legs to go to their upper bodies. Only two parts of your body need to work when you are running—your lungs and your legs.

Sprinting Techniques to Become Faster

To become a faster short distance runner, use the following techniques in your training:

Explosive starts

When you begin running, stay low for the first five to ten yards and lean forward, taking short steps as you accelerate. Do not stand straight up when you begin your sprint. This will slow you down immediately.

The running sprint workouts are 10 to 400 meters in length. After each sprint, walk back to the starting line and begin again. Sprinting activates muscle fibers in your legs that can cause discomfort if not properly stretched and warmed up.

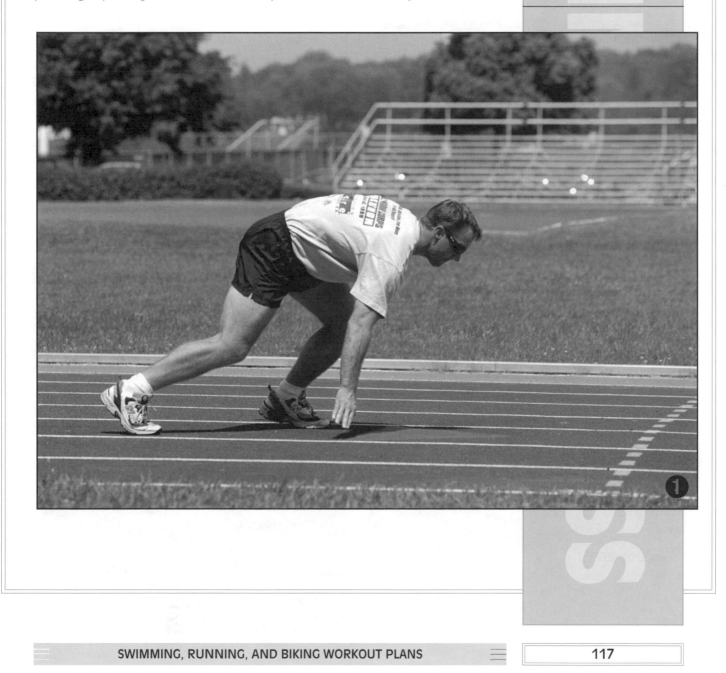

Lean forward and pump those arms

In short distances, such as 20 to 100 yard sprints, leaning forward and pumping your arms quickly will really help increase your speed.

Shift into second gear

After ten yards, it is time to change gears. This is when you will pop up, stick your chest out, pump those arms hard, and lengthen your stride.

Breathing

When you are running as fast as you can, you naturally have to breathe. Your breaths should be quick inhales and quick exhales; unlike like the big, deep breaths you take when you are jogging a few miles.

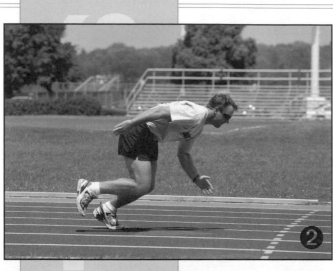

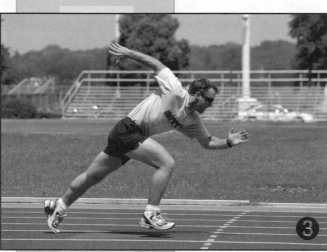

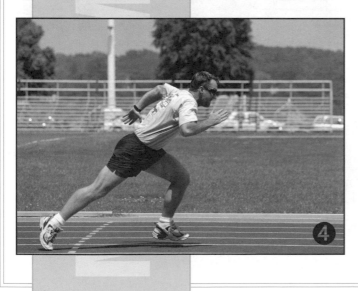

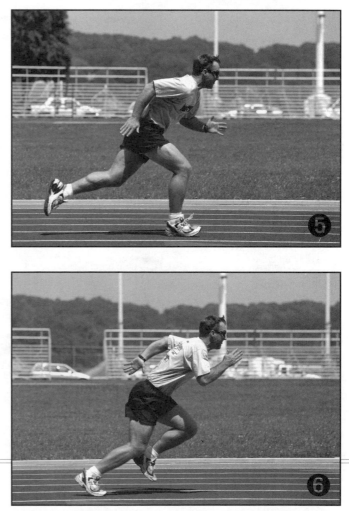

Weight Training Workout Plans

6

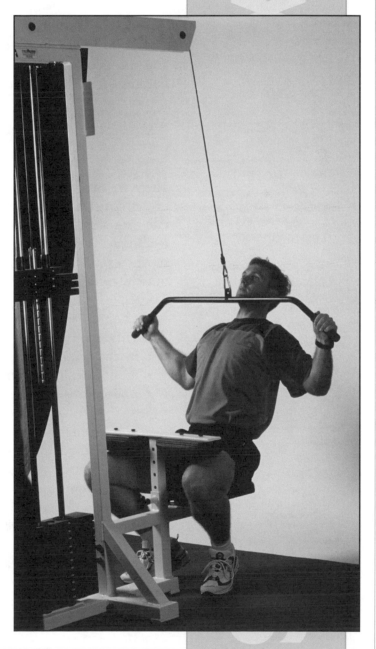

While I was on the football, rugby, and power-lifting teams during high school and college, I lifted heavy weights daily for strength and size. In Navy SEAL training, I rarely lifted heavy weights on a regular basis. However, during cycles such as the winter months on the SEAL Teams, I discovered that a few extra pounds of mass kept me warmer while SCUBA diving in 35- to 45-degree water. Therefore, we developed a workout program to quickly gain weight. Our motto was, " If you want to be big, you have to eat big!" Within a few months, we gained an average of 10 to 15 pounds. *I never took steroids or any supplements, other than a daily multi-vitamin.*

In addition, this workout increased our bench press, squats and lift maximums. Most of the team was able to bench press close to twice their body weight by the end of this program. We discovered that although we did endurance workouts most of the year, weight training was a welcomed rest from the repetition of calisthenics. The hardcore PT cycle and endurance training never affected our strength. In fact, we maintained at least 85 percent of our maximums throughout the year, without lifting a single weight for three-quarters. This test prompted me to write **Maximum Fitness**.

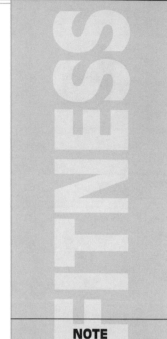

The first two weeks of the power lifting cycle consist of warm-up and PT exercises, combined with heavy weightlifting to track your maximum lifts at the starting point. These first two weeks slowly prepare your muscles for heavier weights, just as the last 13 weeks allow a slow transition into weight training.

Warm Up to Heavy Weights

Weeks 1 and 2

During this transition period, you will lift heavier weights than in the previous 13-week weight/PT cycle. These two weeks will be challenging since you still perform cardiovascular workouts, PT exercises, and heavy weight training—cross training at it's best.

Power lifting Supersets

Weeks 3, 4, and 5

There are two ways to implement a superset, which is a combination of two exercises performed consecutively without any rest. 1) Complete two separate exercises that effect the same muscle group, called the pre-exhaustion technique. The drawback to this technique is that you lose strength for the second exercise. 2) The best way to superset is to pair exercises of opposing muscle groups (antagonist groups). Such muscles groups include:

- Chest & Back
- Thighs & Hamstrings
- Biceps & Triceps
- Front Deltoids & Rear Deltoids
- Abdominals & Lower Back Muscles

When pairing antagonistic exercises, a decrease in strength is avoided. In fact, your strength might increase as blood from the first muscle group used warms the muscles and joints of the opposing muscles being trained. For instance, if you superset dumbbell curls with triceps extensions, blood in your biceps will improve the lifting abilities of your triceps. Therefore, only perform supersets where opposing muscle groups are paired together. Supersets not only allow more work in a shorter period of time, but they improve endurance, increase pump, and help burn fat by elevating the heart rate to the fat-burning zone. The stress created by this technique causes a natural rise in growth hormone levels, which are responsible for fat loss and muscle tissue enhancement.

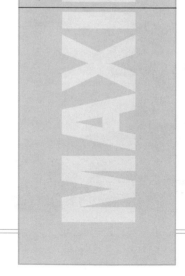

NOTE

Increase the weight of all exercises by five percent each week. For example, if on the fourth week (the first week of the growth phase) you bench press 300 pounds for six to seven reps, then on the fifth week, you bench press 315 pounds (300 x .05=315) for five to six reps. Likewise, on the sixth week you bench press 330 pounds (315 x .05=330.75) for four to five reps.

In the following superset, repeat both exercises for eight sets each:

- Superset
- Incline Dumbbell Bench Press – eight sets of 10 to 12 reps (no rest)
- Close Grip Pull-up (palms facing you) – eight sets of 10 to 12 reps (one-minute rest)

Modified Compound Supersets

Weeks 6, 7, and 8

Modified compound supersets pair antagonist exercises to work opposing muscle groups, with little rest in between. For instance, a chest exercise is followed by a back exercise and brief rest, before repeating the superset. An example of a modified compound superset is incline dumbbell presses paired with dumbbell rows.

MODIFIED SUPERSET: *REPEAT EACH SET FOUR TIMES*

- Incline Dumbbell Presses – one set of 10 to 12 reps
- Rest 60 seconds
- Dumbbell Rows – one set of 10 to 12 reps
- Rest 60 seconds

Each muscles group has a two-minute rest in addition to the time the opposing muscle exercise is performed. The technique of pairing agonistic (same) and antagonists (opposite) muscles in a modified superset not only saves time and keeps the body warm, but provides faster recovery of the nervous system between sets. This enables you to lift heavier weights than if you remained idle for two to three minutes waiting to recover. Training regimens of this nature should last no longer than one hour to an hour and a half.

Week 9 — Rest

During this week, only stretch and perform light cardiovascular exercises to recover from the growth phase and prepare for the power phase.

MAXIMUM FITNESS

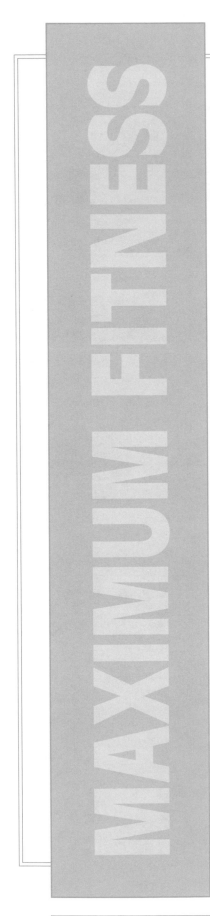

Power Phase Finale

Weeks 10, 11, and 12

Increase the weight of all exercises by five percent each week. For example, if on the tenth week (the first week of the power phase) you bench press 315 pounds for two to four reps, then on the eleventh week, you bench press 330 pounds (315 x .05=330.75) for one to three reps. Likewise, on the twelfth week, you bench press approximately 345 pounds (330 x .05=346.5) for one to two reps.

EXAMPLE:

Day One (Monday/Thursday)
Chest & Back Modified Compound Superset

- Bench Press – eight sets (four, four, three, three, two, two, one, one) of reps with a 150-second rest
- Pulldowns – eight sets (four, four, three, three, two, two, one, one) of reps with a 150-second rest

Mega-Weight/PT Super Burnout Circuit Week

Week 13

Each circuit workout takes approximate 30 minutes to reach total muscle fatigue. Warm up and stretch well before starting each day of exercises. Follow the workouts precisely as you rotate between exercises. Re-read the circuit workout explanations in the weights chapter if unclear.

Workout Charts

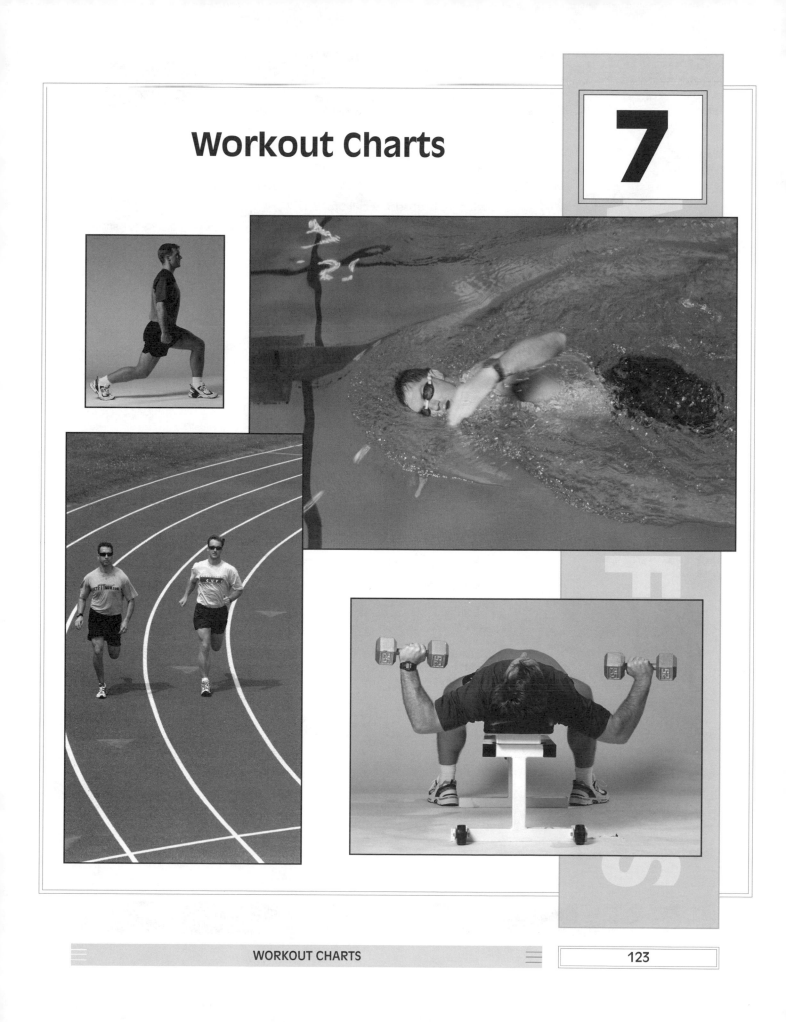

7

Calisthenic Base Cycle: No Weights

MONDAY

UPPER BODY

Push/Pull
  Walk/Run .... 1 mile

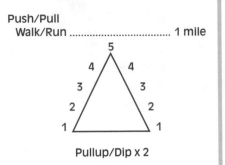

Pullup/Dip x 2

Beginners: Use assisted pull-ups/dips
if needed

Alternating circuit:
Push-ups / Dips / Stomach
Repeat 3 times:
  Reg. Crunches 10
  Push-ups 10
  Rev. Crunches 10
  Chair Dips 10

Stomach exercise: *10 seconds hold
for each rep

TUESDAY

UPPER BODY

Push/Pull
  Walk/Run .... 1 mile
  Pullup/ Dip .... x 2 pyramid

(Beginners: Use assisted pull-ups/dips
if needed)

Alternating circuit:
Pushups / Dips / Stomach
Repeat 3 times:
  Reg. Crunches 10
  Pushups 10
  Rev. Crunches 10

WEDNESDAY

PT DAY OFF
  Stretch 15:00

Stretch routine #1
  (day off stretch)

Run/walk
  Running/walking ...... 20–30 minutes

THURSDAY

UPPER BODY

Push / Pull exercise:
Asst. Pull-ups
Knee Pushup

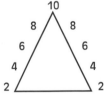

Pull-ups / Push-ups

Dips 10–15
Adv. Crunches .... 10 (1 sec. holds)

Beginners: Use assisted pull-ups/dips,
knee push-ups if needed

Stomach exercises
  Crunches .... 10 x 10 secs
  L/R crunches .... 10 x 10sec
  Side crunches .... 2 x 25
  Rev. Crunches 20

FRIDAY

LOWER BODY

Run/Walk

Repeat 3 times:
  Walk/run 3:00
  1/2 Squats 20
  1/2 Lunges 20/leg
  Heel Raises 30
  Leg stretch 2:00
  thigh
  hamstring
  calves

  Cool down walk/jog 5:00
  Stretch 10:00

SATURDAY

FULL UPPER BODY

Repeat Monday
  Except Bike 20:00 instead of
  walking

Weeks 1–2

Calisthenic Base Cycle: No Weights

MONDAY

UPPER BODY PUSH/PULL DAY

Pushup/Crunch superset:
5 cycles of:
- Regular 5
- Reg. crunch 15
- Wide 5
- Rev. crunch 15
- Tricep 5
- 1/2 situps 15

Pull-ups:
- Regular grip 1,2,3,4,5,6
- Reverse grip 6,5,4,3,2,1
- Assisted pull-ups for beginners

Ab Exercises:
- Reg. Crunches 25
- Rev. Crunches 25
- R. Crunches 25
- L. Crunches 25
- 1/2 situps 25

Pushup / Jumping Jacks superset
Repeat 10x's:
- Jumping jacks 10
- Push-ups 5–10

TUESDAY

LOWER BODY

Run/Walk/Bike .... 20 minutes

Pick one event:
- Squats .... 3 x 20
- Lunges .... 3 x 10
- Calves .... 3 x 25
- Jumping Jacks .... 3 x 20
- Side Crunches .... 4 x 25
- L/R Crunches .... 4 x 25

WEDNESDAY

PT DAY OFF

Stretch 15:00

Stretch routine #1
(day off stretch)

Run/walk
20–30 minutes of running/walking
- Walk .... 20 yds
- Run .... 20 yds
- Repeat for 20–30minutes

THURSDAY

UPPER BODY

Push / Pull exercise
Repeat 5 times: (non-stop)
- Pull-ups 5–10
- Push-ups 10–20
- Crunches .... 10 x 5 seconds
- Dips 10
- Jog .... 1:00 or jumping jacks :30
- (Beginners - assisted pull-ups/dips knee push-ups- if needed)

Biking .... 20 minutes

Ab workout #1
Repeat 2–3 times:
- Reg. Crunches 25
- Rev. Crunches 25
- Alt. reg/rev. crunches ....25 each
- Left leg lever crunches 25
- Right leg lever crunches 25

FRIDAY

NO PT

Stretch .... rest today

Get ready for Saturday full body workout!!

SATURDAY

FULL BODY

- Walk / Run 15:00
- Repeat exercises .... 3 x's
- Push-ups 10–20
- Squats 10–20
- Dips 10–20
- Lunges ... 10–15/leg Crunches 2 x 25 (regular / reverse)
- Heel raises 20
- Pull-ups 10–15
- Crunches .... 2 x 25 (left/right)

3:00 bike or run

Full body Stretch

Week 3

Calisthenic Base Cycle: No Weights

MONDAY

Walk 5:00
Stretch 10:00

FULL BODY

Push / Pull Day
Repeat 3 x's
Push-ups 10
Squats 10
Chair Dips 8
Lunges .... 10 /leg
Pull-ups 10
Calves 10

Repeat abs 2x's

Abs / lower back
Reg. crunches 25
Rev. crunches 25
Left crunches 25
Right crunches 25
Belly flutterkicks 20
R. arm / L. leg lifts 20

TUESDAY

PT DAY OFF

Stretch 15:00
Stretch routine #1 (day off stretch)

Run/walk
Running / walking .... 20–30 minutes

WEDNESDAY

Walk 5:00
Stretch 10:00

UPPER BODY CIRCUIT TRAINING
Repeat 2 x's
Push-ups 10–15
Crunches 20
Lower back #1 20
Pull-ups 15
Rev. crunches 20
Rev. pull-ups 15
Crunches 20
Dips 10
Rev. crunches 20
Lower back #1 10
Crunches 20
Lower back #2 20
Arm Haulers 20
Rev. crunches 20
Lower back #3 20

THURSDAY

Walk 5:00
Stretch 10:00

LEGS /LOVE HANDLES CIRCUIT TRAINING
Repeat 3 x's
Squats 20
L. crunches 20
Lunges 10/leg
R. crunches 20
Heel raise 30
L. crunches 20
*Walk/jog or bike 2:00

Belly flutterkicks .... 2 x 20
R. arm / L. leg lifts .... 2 x 20
Stretch legs 10:00

* Walk/jog/bike around house/
in yard etc. for 2:00 each sets.
Helps loosen the legs

FRIDAY

PT DAY OFF

Stretch 15:00

Stretch routine #1
(day off stretch)

Run/walk
20–30 minutes of running / walking

SATURDAY

Walk 5:00
Stretch 10:00

FULL BODY CIRCUIT
Repeat 2 x's
Push-ups 10–15
Squats 20
Crunches 20
Lower back #1 20
Pull-ups 15
Lunges 10/leg
Rev. crunches 20
Calves .... 25 / leg
Push-ups 10–15
Dips 10
Rev. crunches 20
Lower back #2 10
Squats 20
Arm Haulers 20
Rev. crunches 20
Lunges 10/leg
Crunches 20

Week 4

Calisthenic Base Cycle: No Weights

MONDAY

Walk	5:00
Stretch	10:00
Push-ups	10,10,10
(wide,regular,close)	
Bike or Walk	3:00
Regular crunches	10
(10 second holds)	
Dips	15
Bike or Walk	3:00
Reverse crunches	10
(5 second holds)	
Crunches	4 x 25
Bike or Walk	3:00
Shoulder circles	1:00
(up,front,side, military)	
Belly flutterkicks	2 x 20
R. arm / L. leg lifts	2 x 20
Walk or bike	5:00
Stretch	5:00

TUESDAY

Walk	5:00
Stretch	10:00

LEGS, BACK AND ABS

Alternate Pull-ups/abs	
Pull-ups	3 x 15
(regular or assisted)	
Side crunches	3 x 20
(w/outer thigh lifts)	
Bike or walk	4:00
Alternate pull-ups/abs	
reverse pull-ups	3x 15
Side crunches	3 x 20
(w/inner thigh lifts)	
Bike or walk	4:00
Alternate leg exercise	
Squats	3 x 15
Lunges	3 x 10 / leg
Heel raises	3 x 20
Bike	4:00
Stretch	5:00

WEDNESDAY

PT DAY OFF

Walk	20:00
Stretch	10:00

THURSDAY

New warmup
Repeat 10 times in 5:00:

Jumping jacks	10
Push-ups	5–10

Upper body stretch

Upper body:
Push / Pull exercise

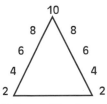

Pull-ups / Push-ups

Repeat 2 times:
Change grip on reverse side of pyramid

FRIDAY

LEG AND LOVEHANDLES

Repeat 4 times:

Bike or walk	5:00
Squats	1:00
Lunges	1:00
Calves	1:00

Love handles
Repeat 3 times:

Side crunches	3 x 25
(w/inner thigh lifts)	
L/R Crunches	3 x 25
Outer thigh leg lifts	25
Swimmers	20
R. arm / L. leg lifts	20

SATURDAY

Jumping jacks/pushup	
Warmup	5:00
Stretch	10:00

CARDIO OPTION DAY

Walk/run	30:00
or Bike	30:00
(see bike workouts)	
or swim	30:00

Or challenge yourself with 2 of the 3 options

Cool down / stretch	10:00

Week 5

Calisthenic Base Cycle: No Weights

MONDAY

Jog/Walk 5:00
Stretch 5:00

Repeat 2x's if too easy

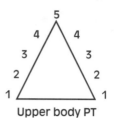

Upper body PT

FULL UPPER BODY
Pull-ups .... x 2
Push-ups .... x 4
Crunches .... x 5
Dips .... x 4
   Beginners: Use assisted dips /
   pull-ups and knee push-ups

Belly flutterkicks 20
R. arm / L. leg lifts 20

Jog/bike 20:00

Stretch

TUESDAY

Warmup .... repeat 10x's
Jumping jacks 10
½ Squats 10

LOWER BODY—ABS
Squats .... 3 x 20
L/R crunches .... 3 x 40
Run/bike 3:00
Lunges .... 3 x 10/leg
L/R crunches .... 3 x 40
Run/Bike 3:00
Calves .... 3 x 25
Side crunches .... x 40

Run / Bike 3:00

Belly flutterkicks 20
R. arm / L. leg lifts 20

Stretch 5:00

WEDNESDAY

PT DAY OFF
jog/walk 20:00
Stretch 10:00

THURSDAY

Warmup .... repeat 10x's
Jumping jacks 10
Push-ups 10
   Repeat 5–10 times

UPPER BODY PUSH / ABS
Wide push-ups 5–10
Reg. Crunches 20
Reg. Push-ups 5–10
Rev. Crunches 20
Tricep push-ups 5–10
½ Situps 20

Belly flutterkicks 20
R. arm / L. leg lifts 20

Jog/bike 20:00

Stretch

FRIDAY

Jog/ Walk 5:00
Stretch 5:00
   Repeat 4 times

LEGS AND BACK
Belly flutterkicks 20
R. arm / L. leg lifts 20
Squats .... 20 reps
Lunges .... 10 reps
Calves .... 20 reps
L/R crunches 25
Side crunches 25
   (both sides on abs)

Jog/bike 20:00

Stretch

SATURDAY

Repeat 5–10 x's
   Jumping jacks 10
   Pushup 5–10
   Stretch 10:00

UPPER BODY CIRCUIT
Repeat 3 x's
Push-ups 15
Crunches 20
Lower back #1 20
Pull-ups 10–15
Rev. crunches 20
Wide Push-ups 10–15
Dips 10–15
Rev. crunches 20
Lower back #2 10
Arm Haulers 20
Rev. pull-ups 10–15
Rev. crunches 20
Crunches 20

*Use knee push-ups, assisted dips
and pull-ups if needed

Weeks 6–8

Rest Week

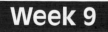

Calisthenic Base Cycle: No Weights

MONDAY

Warmup .... repeat 5–10x's
Jumping jacks 10
Push-ups 10

UPPER BODY PT

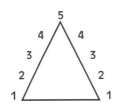

1. Pull-ups .... x 1
2. Push-ups .... x 2
3. Abs .... x 3
4. Dips .... x 2

TUESDAY

Warmup .... repeat 10x's
Jumping jacks 10
½ Squats 10

LEG / AB WORKOUT
Repeat 3–4 times
  Squats 20
  Lunges 20
  Calf raise 25
  Side crunches .... 25 each side

BIKE
  push / pull peddle .... 1:00 / 1:00
    for 20–30 minutes
  push 1:00
  pull 1:00
    alternating every 1:00
    (need straps for feet to pull)

WEDNESDAY

Warmup .... repeat 5–10x's
Jumping jacks 10
Push-ups 10

REVERSE PYRAMID

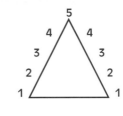

CHEST / ABS
  25–1 push-ups
  50–2 crunches of choice
  1st set ... 25 push-ups / 50 crunches
  2nd set .. 24 push-ups / 48 crunches
  3rd set ... 23 push-ups / 46 crunches
    all the way to 1 on push-ups and
    2 on abs
  25 total sets

  Jog/bike .... 20 minutes
  Stretch

THURSDAY

Warmup .... repeat 5-10's
Jumping jacks 10
Stretch ...... 15 seconds each stretch

UPPER BODY
Repeat 2 times
  50 pull-ups in as few sets as
  possible
  (do assisted if needed)

Ab day-off

  Jog/bike 20:00
  Stretch

FRIDAY

Warmup .... repeat 10x's
Jumping jacks 10
½ Squats 10

LEG SUPERSET
Repeat 2–3 times
  Jog/walk ....1/2 mile
  Squats 20
  1/2 squats 20
  4-count squats 10
  Walking squats 10/side
  Lunges 10-20/leg
  Walking lunges 20steps
  Calves regular 20
  Calves - toe in 20
  Calves - toe out 20
  Calves - bent knee 20

  Stretch 3:00

SATURDAY

Repeat .... 5–10x's
Jumping jacks 10
Pushup 5–10
Stretch 10:00

UPPER BODY PT CIRCUIT
Repeat 2 times (no rest)
  Pull-ups .... max + 3negs
  Abs .... max in 2:00
  Dips .... max + 3 negs
  Abs .... max in 2:00
  Push-ups .... max in 2:00
  Abs .... max in 2:00

  Jog/bike 20:00

  Stretch

Weeks 10–12

12

Calisthenic Base Cycle: No Weights

MONDAY

Warmup .... repeat 5–10x's
Jumping jacks 10
Push-ups 10

SPARTAN RUN
Run 1 mile
   100 push-ups
   100 abs of choice
Run 1 mile
   75 push-ups
   75 abs of choice
Run 1 mile
   50 push-ups
   50 abs of choice

(Do PT in as few sets as possible)

TUESDAY

Warmup .... repeat 10x's
Jumping jacks 10
½ Squats 10

LEG /BIKE PT
Repeat 4 times
   Squats 1:00
   Walking lunges 1:00
   Calves 1:00
   Bike 3:00

WEDNESDAY

Warmup .... repeat 5–10x's
Jumping jacks 10
Push-ups 10

MEGA-MAX WORKOUT

	Pull-ups	Push-ups	Dips
1.	max	max	max
2.	max-2	max-10	max-4
3.	max-4	max-20	max-8
4.	max-6	max-30	max-2
5.	max-8	max-40	max-6

(no rest -from exercise to exercise)

Sprint / Run
50 yd sprint / 50 yd jog
for 10, 20 , 30 minutes

THURSDAY

Warmup .... repeat 5–10's
Jumping jacks 10
Stretch ...... 15 seconds each stretch

UPPER BODY

Bike / Lifecycle pyramid
   Level 1-12-1
      1:00 each level (manual mode)
      Total time: 23 minutes

Bike
Push / pull peddle
   1:00 / 1:00 .... 20–30 minutes
   Push 1:00
   Pull 1:00
      Alternating every 1:00
      (need straps for feet to pull)

FRIDAY

Warmup .... repeat 10x's
Jumping jacks 10
½ Squats 10

LEG SUPERSET
Repeat 3 times
   Jog/walk ....1/4 mile
   Squats 20
   1/2 squats 20
   4-count squats 10
   Walking squats 10/side

   Jog/walk ....1/4 mile
   Lunges 10–20/leg
   Walking lunges .... 20 steps

   Jog/walk ....1/4 mile
   Calves regular 20
   Calves - toe in 20
   Calves - toe out 20
   Calves - bent knee 20
   Stretch 3:00

SATURDAY

Repeat .... 5–10x's
Jumping jacks 10
Pushup 5–10

Swim / PT
Repeat 10 times
   Swim (choice) 100m
   Push-ups 10–20
   Abs of choice 20
   Pullouts 5

AND / OR

Sprint / PT
Repeat 10 times
   Pull-ups 10
   Push-ups 20
   Abs of choice 30
   Run 100yds

   Stretch 10:00

Week 13

Hardcore PT: Run, Swim, Bike

MONDAY

Warmup/Stretch

UPPER BODY—PUSH/PULL DAY

PT PYRAMID
- Pull-ups 1-10-1
- Push-ups 2-20-2
- Abs of choice 5-50-5

Running
3 mile track workout
- Jog .... 1 mile in 7:00-8:00
- Sprint .... 1/4 mile
- Jog .... 1/4 mile in 2:00
- Sprint .... 1/4 mile in
- Jog .... 1/4 mile in 2:00
- Sprint ....1/8 mile
- Jog .... 1/8 mile in 1:00
- Sprint ....1/8 mile
- Jog .... 1/8 mile in 1:00
- Sprint ....1/8 mile
- Jog .... 1/8 mile in 1:00
- Sprint ....1/8 mile
- Jog .... 1/8 mile in 1:00

TUESDAY

Warmup/Stretch

LOWER BODY

Bike (or jog) mixed with leg PT
Repeat 3 times
- Bike 5:00
- Squats 1:00
- Lunges 1:00
- Calves 1:00
- Abs max 2:00*
  - *abs - can be your choice of:
    situps, 1/2 situps or crunches

- Swim 1000m
- Swim .... 500m with fins
- Swim .... 500m without fins
  stroke of choice
  side or freestyle stroke

Cool down / Stretch

WEDNESDAY

Warmup/Stretch

SWIM /RUN /BIKE DAY

Swim sprints
Repeat 10 times:
- sprint 100m
- 50m slow (catch breath)
  (1500m total)

Abs Love handles
Repeat 4 times:
- Side-crunches .... 25 / side
- Lower back flutters 20sec

Bike (lifecycle pyramid)
- Level 1-12-1
- 1:00 each level of pyramid
  (manual mode)
  total time: 23 minutes

or Running workout

Cool down / Stretch

THURSDAY

Warmup/Stretch

UPPER BODY

Push / Pull exercise
Repeat 10 times:
- Jumping jacks 10
- Push-ups 10

Upper body PT
10 Supersets
- Pull-ups 8
- Push-ups 20
- Abs of choice 20
- Dips 10

Cool down / Stretch

FRIDAY

Warmup/Stretch

LOWER BODY—RUN/WALK

Running / Leg PT
- Jog .... 1 mile
- Sprint ....1/4 mile
- Squats 20
- Lunges .... 10 /leg
- Jog .... 1/4 mile in 2:00
- Sprint ....1/4 mile
- Squats 20
- Lunges .... 10 /leg
- Jog .... 1/4 mile in 2:00
- Sprint ....1/8 mile
- Squats 20
- Lunges .... 10 /leg
- Jog .... 1/8 mile in 1:00
- Sprint ....1/8 mile
- Squats 20
- Lunges 10/leg
- Jog .... 1/8 mile in 1:00

No abs today

SATURDAY

Warmup/Stretch

FULL UPPER BODY

Repeat 10 times:
- Jumping jacks 10
- Push-ups 10
  50 pull-ups in as few sets as
  possible (goal 2-3)

Swim / pt
Repeat 5-10 times:
- Sprint 100m
- Push-ups 10–20
- Abs of choice 20–30

Cool down / Stretch

Weeks 1–2

Hardcore PT: Run, Swim, Bike

MONDAY

Warmup/Stretch

FULL BODY CIRCUIT
Repeat 3 times
   Jumping jacks 10–20
   Pull-ups ....max
   Push-ups 10–20
   Squats w/heel raise 20–30
     Repeat 3 times
   Jumping jacks 10–20
   Pull-ups 5–10
   Dips 10–20
   Lunges .... 10–20 per leg
     Repeat 3 times
   Jumping jacks 10–20
   Tricep push-ups 10–20
   Pull-ups 5–10
     Repeat 4 times

TUESDAY

Warmup/Stretch

RUN-SWIM-RUN
  1. Run ....2 miles
  2. Swim .... 1000m with or w/o fins
  3. Run ....2 miles

Cool down / Stretch

WEDNESDAY

Warmup/Stretch

LEG / ABS / RUN DAY
Spartan run
   Run .... 1 mile
   Squats with heel raise 50
   Abs of choice 100
   Run .... 1 mile
   Walking lunges .... 40 steps
   Abs of choice 75
   Run .... 1 mile
   Squats w/heel raises 30
   Steps - walking lunges 20
   Abs of choice 50

Cool down / Stretch

THURSDAY

Warmup/Stretch

SWIM PT—UPPER BODY
Push / Pull exercise
   Repeat 10 times .... 100 yards
   Pullouts 5
   Push-ups 10–20
   Abs 20–30

Cool down / Stretch

FRIDAY

Warmup/Stretch

LOWER BODY—BIKE / RUN OR WALK
Repeat 3 times .... total 30 minutes
   *Bike, walk or run 5:00
   Squats 1:00
   Lunges 1:00
   Calves 1:00
   Reg./rev. crunch 1:00
   Stretch legs 1:00
     * best with lifecycle

NO ABS TODAY

Cool down / Stretch

SATURDAY

Warmup/Stretch

FULL UPPER BODY
10–20 minutes of:
   Sprint .... 50 yds
   Jog or walk .... 50 yds

SPRINTS
   20m ....1/2 pace x 2
   20m .... full sprint x 3
   40m ....3/4 pace x 2
   40m ....full sprint x 3
   60m ....full sprint x 5
   80m ....full sprint x 3
   100m ....full sprint x 3
     (rest = walk back to starting line)

PT PYRAMID
   Pull-ups 1-10-1
   Push-ups 3-30-3
   Abs of choice5-50-5

Week 3

Hardcore PT: Run, Swim, Bike

MONDAY

Warmup/Stretch

UPPER BODY—RUN, SWIM

Run - swim /pt - run
1. Run .... 3 miles (18–24:00)
2. Repeat 10 times
Swim 100m
Abs of choice 20
Push-ups 10–20
Pullouts 5

3. Run .... 3 miles (20–24:00)

Cool down / Stretch

TUESDAY

Warmup/Stretch

BIKE / LOWER BODY
Repeat 4 times
Bike 3:00
Squats 1:00
Lunges 1:00
Calves 1:00

Stretch

Cool down / Stretch

WEDNESDAY

Warmup/Stretch

UPPER BODY PT /RUN

Spartan run
Run .... 1 mile
Push-ups (fewest sets) 100
Abs of choice 100

Run .... 1 mile
Push-ups 75
Abs of choice 75

Run .... 1 mile
Push-ups 50
Abs of choice 50

Cool down / Stretch

THURSDAY

Warmup/Stretch

LOWER BODY—SWIM OR WALK

Swim sprints / legs
400m warmup / stretch
200m x 2 ....400m
(100m flutterlicks)
(100m breast kick only)
Squats .... 30 x 2
100m x 4 ....400m
Lunges .... 10 /leg x 4

Just swim
50m x 10 ....500m
25m x 12 ....300m
Total .... 2000 total yards

Cool down / Stretch

FRIDAY

Warmup/Stretch

UPPER BODY—PT WITH THE CLOCK

Alternate each set with:
1:00 x 2 .... situps 50–60
1:00 x 2 .... pushup max

::30 x 4 .... situps 25–30
::30 x 4 .... pushup max

::15 x 4 .... situps-10–15
::15 x 4 .... pushup max

PFT techniques: pace the situps,
sprint the push-ups

No run or swim

Cool down / Stretch

SATURDAY

Warmup/Stretch

SATURDAY TRIATHLON WORKOUT

Swim .... 1 mile
Bike ride ....20 miles
Run ....5 miles

Cool down / Stretch

Week 4

Hardcore PT: Run, Swim, Bike

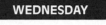

MONDAY

Warmup/Stretch

FULL BODY

Pushup/Crunch—superset:
15 cycles of:
Regular pushup 10
Reg. crunch 10
Wide pushup 10
Rev. crunch 10
Tricep pushup 10
L/R crunches .... 10 / 10

Leg / ab workout
Repeat 3–4 times:
Squats 20
Lunges 20
Heel raise 25
Crunches 50

TUESDAY

Warmup/Stretch

CARDIO

Running
4 Mile Track Work
Jog .... 1 mile in 7:00
Three sets of:
Sprint .... 1/4 mile in
Jog .... 1/4 mile in 1:45
Six sets of:
Sprint .... 1/8 mile
Jog .... 1/8 mile 1:00

Swimming
Hypoxic pyramids

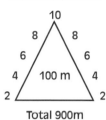

Total 900m

Cool down / Stretch

WEDNESDAY

Warmup/Stretch

FULL BODY

Upper body PT Pull-ups:
Each type of pullup for 5 sets
of 2, 4, 6, 8, 10
1. Regular grip
2. Reverse grip
3. Close grip
4. Wide grip
5. Mountain
climber

pull-ups

10 Supersets
Situps 10
Push-ups 10
Atomic situps 10
Triceps push-ups 10
Leg levers 10
Wide push-ups 10

LEG /BIKE PT
Repeat 4 times
1/2 squats 1:00

THURSDAY

Warmup/Stretch

CARDIO

Run - Sprint - Run
Run .... 2 miles
Sprint .... 1 mile
Run .... 2 miles

Cool down / Stretch

FRIDAY

Warmup/Stretch

UPPER BODY

Mega-MAX workout
1. Pull-ups
2. Push-ups
3. Dips
Max out all 1,2,3
Max-2, max-10, max-4
Max-4, max-20, max-8
Max-6, max-30, max-12
Max-8, max-40, max-16

No rest -exercise to exercise

Object is to max out on all the
exercises on the first set. On the 2nd
set, subtract 2 from your max from
pull-ups, subtract 10 from your max
on push-ups, and subtract 4 from
your max on dips. That is your goal
for set #2 and so on. Each set gets
"easier" on paper, but the goal is
total upper body muscle failure.

Cool down / Stretch

SATURDAY

Warmup/Stretch

FROGMAN—TRIATHLON

Swim w/fins .... 1 mile
Bike ride .... 20 miles
Run in sand on beach .... 5 miles
(if possible)

Cool down / Stretch

Week 5

MONDAY

Warmup/Stretch

UPPER BODY—PUSH/PULL DAY

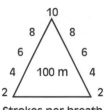

Strokes per breath

In between each 100m hypoxic swim do the following PT:
Pullouts 5
Push-ups 15–20
Abs of choice 20
Run .... 3–5 miles

Cool down / Stretch

TUESDAY

Warmup/Stretch

LOWER BODY

Bike / Leg workout
  Push / pull peddles
  Alternate
  Push 1:00
  1:00 pull 20–30:00
    alternating every 1:00
    (need straps for feet to pull)

Bike / leg PT
Repeat 3 times
  Bike 5:00
  Squats w/heel raise 1:00
  Lunges 1:00
  Calves 1:00
  Abs max 2:00

Cool down / Stretch

WEDNESDAY

Warmup/Stretch

RUN-SWIM-RUN
  1. Run - 3 miles
  2. Swim-1500m w/fins
  3. Run - 3 miles

Cool down / Stretch

THURSDAY

Warmup/Stretch

UPPER BODY
Reverse pyramid
  Chest / abs
  Push-ups 25–1
  Abs of choice 50–2

```
        10
      8    8
    6        6
  4  pull-ups  4
2              2
   Three grips
```

Start with push-ups 25, 24, 23
Alternate with abs 50, 48, 46
  basically double your reps for abs

Pullup pyramid
  1. Regular grip
  2. Reverse grip
  3. Grip of choice
  Total .... 150 pull-ups

Cool down / Stretch

FRIDAY

Warmup/Stretch

LOWER BODY

Track workout—Repeat 3–4 times
  Sprint .... 1 mile
  Walk ....1/2 mile
    (or jog if you can instead of walk)

Sprints
  Sprint x 10 ....10m
  Sprint x 5 ....20m
  Sprint x 5 ....40m
  Sprint x 4 ....60m
  Sprint x 3 ....100m
    (rest = walk to starting line)

Leg PT—Repeat 4 times
  Squats 25
  Lunges 25
  Heel Raise 30

Love Handles
  Side crunches .... 4 x 25
  R/L crunches .... 2 x 50

Cool down / Stretch

SATURDAY

Warmup/Stretch

UPPER BODY

PT with the clock
  Alternate each set:
  Pt max in 2:00 each:
  Max pull-ups ....
  Max push-ups ....
  Max situps ....
  Max dips ....

Repeat 2 times:
  Situps 50–60 in 1:00
  Push-ups max in 1:00
  Situps 25–30 in .... ::30
  Push-ups max in .... ::30
  Situps 10-15 .... ::15
  Push-ups max in .... ::15

PFT techniques : pace the situps not the push-ups

Swim
  1000m with or w/o fins

Cool down / Stretch

Rest Week

Hardcore PT: Run, Swim, Bike

MONDAY

Warmup/Stretch

UPPER BODY—PUSH/PULL DAY

```
          10
       8      8
     6 / dips \ 6
    4 / pull-ups \ 4
   2              2
```
Four grips

Pullup pyramid
1. Regular grip
2. Reverse grip
3. Close grip
4. Grip of choice
Total .... 200 pull-ups

But alternating dips either parallel
bar dips or bench dips
total .... 200 dips

Run
  Timed run .... 4 miles

Cool down / Stretch

TUESDAY

Warmup/Stretch

LOWER BODY

Bike / leg PT
Repeat 4 times:
  Bike 5:00
  Squats 1:00
  Lunges 1:00
  Calves 1:00
  Max situps in 2:00

  Swim with fins 1500m

Cool down / Stretch

WEDNESDAY

Warmup/Stretch

RUN-HYPOXIC SWIM-RUN
  Run .... 3 miles

Hypoxic pyramid

```
          10
       8      8
     6 / dips \ 6
    4 / pull-ups \ 4
   2              2
```
Strokes per breath

  Run .... 3 miles

Cool down / Stretch

THURSDAY

Warmup/Stretch

UPPER BODY

Push / Pull exercise
Repeat 20 times:
  Jumping jacks 10
  Push-ups 10

Swim PT
Repeat 15 times:
  Sprint .... 100 m
  Pullouts 10
  Abs of choice 20–30

Cool down / Stretch

FRIDAY

Warmup/Stretch

LOWER BODY—RUN/WALK

Run / LegPT / Run
  Run .... 2 miles

then . . . Repeat 4 times:
  Walking squats 25yd
  Walking lunges .... 25 yd
  Run .... 1/4 mile

then again . . .
  Run .... 2 miles

Cool down / Stretch

SATURDAY

Warmup/Stretch

FULL UPPER BODY
```
          10
       8      8
     6 / dips \ 6
    4 / pull-ups \ 4
   2              2
```
Four grips

Pullup pyramid
1. Regular grip
2. Reverse grip
3. Close grip
4. Grip of choice
Total .... 200 pull-ups

But alternating push-ups
  Try to double the push-ups on
the   pyramid
total .... 400 push-ups

Swim (with or without fins) ... 2000m

Cool down / Stretch

Weeks 10–12

Hardcore PT: Run, Swim, Bike

MONDAY

Warmup/Stretch

UPPER BODY—PUSH/PULL DAY

Run - Swim /pt - Run
1. Run 5 miles
2. Repeat 15 times
Swim 100m
Abs of choice 20
Push-ups 20
Pullouts 5

3. Run ....5 miles

You can split any of these workouts throughout the day IF you do not have time to do all at once.

Cool down / Stretch

TUESDAY

Warmup/Stretch

LOWER BODY

Running / Leg PT
Jog .... 1 mile
Sprint ....1/4 mile
Squats 40
Lunges .... 20 /leg
Jog .... 1/4 mile in 2:00
Sprint ....1/4 mile
Squats 40
Lunges .... 20 /leg
Jog .... 1/4 mile in 2:00
Sprint ....1/8 mile
Squats 40
Lunges .... 20 /leg
Jog .... 1/8 mile in 1:00
Sprint ....1/8 mile
Squats 40
Lunges 20/leg
Jog .... 1/8 mile in 1:00

Swim with fins
With fins 1000m
Without fins 500m

WEDNESDAY

Warmup/Stretch

UPPER BODY PUSH

25 Supersets
Situps 10
Push-ups 10
Regular Crunches 10
Tricep push-ups 10
Reverse crunches 10
Dips 10
Total time .... 50 minutes

Bike—Lifecycle pyramid
Levels 1-15-1
1:00 each level
(manual mode)
Total time .... 29 minutes

Cool down / Stretch

THURSDAY

Warmup/Stretch

UPPER BODY PULL
Pull-ups .... 250 pull-ups

2,4,6,8,10,8,6,4,2
1. Regular grip
2. Reverse grip
3. Close grip
4. Wide grip
5. Mountain climber

Cool down / Stretch

FRIDAY

Warmup/Stretch

LEG PT—RUN / SWIM WITH FINS

Running
4 Mile Track Workout
Jog .... 1 mile in 7:00

Three sets of:
Sprint .... 1/4 mile in
Jog .... 1/4 mile in 1:45
Squats/calves 30
Lunges 20/leg

Six sets of:
Sprint ....1/8 mile
Jog .... 1/8 mile 1:00

Swim with fins 1000m

Cool down / Stretch

SATURDAY

Warmup/Stretch

FULL UPPER BODY

Repeat 20 times
Jumping jacks 10
Push-ups 10

100 pull-ups in as few sets as possible (goal 4–8)
Rest 2:00 in between each set

BUT . . . 2:00 of max situps is your rest for every set you have to do.

Cool down / Stretch

Week 13

Weights / PT / Cardio Mix

MONDAY

Warmup/Stretch

UPPER BODY—BACK, BI, CHEST, TRI

PT pyramid
Pull-ups 1-10-1
Bench press 2-20-2
   (light weight)
Abs of choice 3-30-3

Back and Biceps
Bent over rows .... 3 x 10
Strip workout . (3 tens on each side)
Curls .... max, strip 1 ten /side
Curls ...... max again, strip 1 ten/side
Curls .... max, strip, max bar
   (at least 50 reps total)

TUESDAY

Warmup/Stretch

LEGS/SHOULDERS—BIKE (OR JOG)

Mixed with leg PT
Repeat 3 times:
   Bike 5:00
   Squats w/weight 30
   Lunges w/weight 10
   Calves w/weight 30
   Crunches 50

Mega Shoulder workout x 1
(1,2 or 5 lbs DB's)
   Lateral raises 10
   Lat raises (thumb up) 10
   Lat raise #3 10
     (thumbs up/down)
   Front raise 10
   Front raise ..... 10 (thumb up/down)
   Cross over jacks 10
   Military press 10

Swim

WEDNESDAY

Warmup/Stretch

LIGHT CARDIO DAY

Swim sprints
Repeat 5 times:
   Sprint 100m
   Slow (catch breath) 50m
   (750m total)

Abs - Super set
Repeat 4 times:
   Side-crunches .... 25 / side
   Lower back flutters 20sec
   10 second crunch 10
   Reg/rev. crunch 25
     (alternate reg./rev. crunch)
   Abs stretch

Bike (lifecycle pyramid)
   Level 1-12-1
   Each level of pyramid 1:00
     (manual mode)
   Total time .... 23 minutes

Cool down / Stretch

THURSDAY

Warmup/Stretch

UPPER BODY—BACK, BI, CHEST, TRI

Upper body weight / PT Circuit
workout
   Pull-ups .... max + 3 negs
   Dips .... max + 3 negatives
   Abs .... max in 2:00
   Bench press .... 50% max
     (max + 3 negatives)
   Push-ups .... max in 1:00
   Pulldowns .... 50% bodyweight
     (max + 3 negatives)
   Abs .... max in 2:00
   Military press .... max reps
     (dumbells 20–30lbs)
   Bicep curls .... max reps (20–30lbs)
   Tri ext .... max reps (20lbs)
   Abs .... max in 2:00

Repeat 10 times

FRIDAY

Warmup/Stretch

RUN
   Run .... 3-5 miles

Cool down / Stretch

SATURDAY

Warmup/Stretch

BACK, BI, LEGS

Back / leg
   Repeat 2-3 times
   Squats 30
   Pull-ups 10, 8, 6, 4, 2
     15sec rest in between
   Leg ext .... 10, 15, 20 reps
     (decreasing weight)
   Leg curls 10, 15, 20
     (decreasing weight)
   Lunges .... 30 steps
   Bent over rows 20-15-10
   Calves 25
   Calves, bent knee 25

*Weights are different for every-
one. You should try to lift enough
weight so the reps suggested are
just possible.

Cool down / Stretch

Week 1–2

Weights / PT / Cardio Mix

MONDAY

Warmup/Stretch

CHEST, TRI, SHOULDERS

Repeat 5 times:
Jumping jacks 10
Push-ups 10
Bench .... 75% max 3 x max
Incline DB .... 3 x 10
  (rest with 25 abs in between sets)
DB flies .... 3 x 10
  (alt. abs)
Abs of choice .... 3 x 25
Push-ups .... max in 2:00
Tri push-ups .... 3 x 15
Close bench .... 3 x 10
Tri ext .... 3 x 15 (DB)
Tri kickbacks .... 3 x 10
Military .... 3 x 15
Upright rows .... 3 x 10
  (alt w/ push-ups
Push-ups .... 3 x 10

Three sets of the Mega-shoulder
workout: 5 lbs, 2 lbs, and no weight

jog/bike 15:00–30:00

TUESDAY

Warmup/Stretch

BACK, BI'S, LEGS

Repeat 10 times:
Jumping jacks 10
Squats 10

Repeat 2 times:
Squats .... 30 w / weight
Leg ext .... 10, 15, 20 reps
  (decreasing weight)
Leg curls 10,15,20
  (decreasing weight)
Lunges .... 30 steps

Back / Biceps
Max pull-ups +3 negs
Wide pulldowns .... 3 x 10
Reg. pulldowns .... 3 x 10
Rev. pulldowns .... 3 x 10

Dumbell PT .... 3x's

WEDNESDAY

Warmup/Stretch

SWIM / RUN DAY

Run .... 2 miles
Swim 1000m

Cool down / Stretch

THURSDAY

Warmup/Stretch

FULL BODY CIRCUIT

Full body weight / PT circuit
Repeat 2–3 times
Pull-ups 5–15
Push-ups 10–20
Squats w/heel raise 20–30
Dips 10–20
Lunges 10–15/leg
Crunches .... 50 of your choice
Side crunches 25/side
Lower back flutters .... 30 seconds
Military press 10–15
Bicep curls 10–20
Tricep ext 10–20
Hammer curls 10–20
1/2 situps .... max in 2:00

Sprints (rest: walk back to starting line)
20m ....1/2 pace x 2
20m ....full sprint x 3
40m ....3/4 pace x 2
40m ....full sprint x 3
60m ....full sprint x 5
80m ....full sprint x 3
100m ....full sprint x 3

FRIDAY

REST DAY

Stretch

SATURDAY

Warmup/Stretch

FULL BODY

19 mintues workout
  (light weights for max reps)
Bench press 1:00
Squats 1:00
Pulldowns 1:00
Bike / jog 3:00
Military press 1:00
Lunges .... 30 seconds each leg
Bicep curls 1:00
Bike 3:00
Tricep ext 1:00
Heel raises 1:00
Leg ext 1:00
Leg curls 1:00
Bike 3:00

Try it two times if you were not
challenged.

Week 3

Weights / PT / Cardio Mix

MONDAY

Warmup/Stretch

CHEST, TRI, SHOULDERS

Run - swim /pt - run
1. Run ....2 miles
2. Repeat 10 times
Swim 100m
Abs of choice 20
Push-ups 10–20
Pullouts 5
3. Run ....2 miles
Bench Press 10, 8, 6, 4, 2, 1
Incline press .... 3 x 10
Dips .... 3 x 15-20
Tricep ext .... 3 x 10
Pushdowns .... 3 x 15
Abs superset .... x 2
Reg. crunch 25
Rev. crunch 25
L/R crunch .... 25 / side
1/2 situps 25
Side crunch .... 25 each side

Mega shoulder workout
1,2 or 5 lbs dumbbells
lateral raises 10

TUESDAY

Warmup/Stretch

BIKE / BICEPS LEGS & ABS
Repeat 3 times
Bike or run 5:00
Squats 1:00
Lunges 1:00
Calves 1:00
Situps .... max in 2:00
  or crunches

Repeat 3 times
Legs with dumbells
Squats w/heel raises 20
Lunges .... 15 /leg
Side crunches 25/side
Bike 4:00
Bicep curls 15
Leg ext 20
Leg curls 20
Hammer curls 15
Bike 4:00

Stretch
Cool down / Stretch

WEDNESDAY

Warmup/Stretch

HYPOXIC SWIM DAY

Warmup 100m
100m x 9 sets 900m
Total...............................1000m

Cool down / Stretch

THURSDAY

Warmup/Stretch

FULL BODY CIRCUIT
25,20,15 circuit of reps
(alternate each exercise)
Bench press 25, 20, 15
Military press 25, 20, 15
Squats w/ heel raises 25, 20, 15
Lunges .... 25, 20, 15 / leg
Pulldowns or pull-ups 25, 20, 15
Leg ext 25, 20, 15
Pushdowns 25, 20, 15
Leg curls 25, 20, 15
Bicep curls 25, 20, 15
Tricep ext 25, 20, 15
Bent knee heel raise 25, 20, 15
L/R/reg./reverse crunches ..... 4 x 25
Bike / jog 5:00

*Go through circuit . . . 1st circuit is
25 each, 2nd rotation is 20 each
exercise, and 3rd rotation is 15
each exercise. Non-stop -no rest.

Cool down / Stretch

FRIDAY

Warmup/Stretch

SWIM DAY
400m warmup/ stretch
Flutterlicks 100m
Breast kick 100m
100m x 4 ....400m
50m x 10 ....500m
25m x 12 ....300m
Total................................1800m

Cool down / Stretch

SATURDAY

Warmup/Stretch

SATURDAY TRIATHLON WORKOUT

Swim .... 1 mile
Bike ride ....20 miles
Run ....5 miles

Cool down / Stretch

Week 4

Weights / PT / Cardio Mix

MONDAY

Warmup/Stretch

MAX UPPER BODY

Repeat 3 times:
Jumping jacks 10
Push-ups 10

Bench press .... *Two pops
Pull-ups .... max
Situps .... max in 2:00
Push-ups .... max in 2:00
Pulldowns .. max reps of 75% bdywt

*Two pops refer to the number of
reps done per set as you increase
the weight each set. Only do two
reps for the first four sets, then
just do one rep until unable to
increase the weight.

**Use spotter at all times.

Swim .... 500m freestyle

Cool down / Stretch

TUESDAY

Warmup/Stretch

MAX LOWER BODY
Repeat 3 times:
Jumping jacks 10
Squats 10
Squats .... 5 x 5 reps
   (increasing weight)
Leg curls .... 5 x 5 reps
   (increasing weight)
Leg ext .... 5 x 5 reps
   (increasing weight each set)
Run ....2 miles

Ab workout #1
Repeat 2–3 times:
Reg. Crunches 25
Rev. Crunches 25
Alt. reg./rev crunches ....25 each
Left leg lever crunches 25
Right leg lever crunches 25

Cool down / Stretch

WEDNESDAY

Warmup/Stretch

BACK, BI, SHOULDERS:
   Each type of pullup
   for 4 sets of 2, 4, 6, 8, 10
   1. Regular grip
   2. Reverse grip
   3. Close grip
   4. Wide grip

Dumbell PT: 3x's
Reverse Flies 15
Upright Rows- 15
Shrugs 15
Lateral raises 15
Lawnmowers 15
Bicep Curls 15

MEGA SHOULDER WORKOUT
1, 2 or 5 lbs dumbbells
Love Handles .... repeat 3 times
Side Oblique .... 25 each side
Inner-OuterThigh crunch 25
   (both sides and legs = 100)

Cool down / Stretch

THURSDAY

Warmup/Stretch

CARDIO
   Run – Sprint – Run
   Run ....2 miles
   Sprint .... 1 mile
   Run ....2 miles

Lower / Upper Back
   Lower Back # 1 25
   Lower back ex #2 25
   Swimmers 25
   Reverse push-ups 25
   Arm Haulers 25

Cool down / Stretch

FRIDAY

Warmup/Stretch

UPPER BODY

Mega-MAX workout
   1. Pull-ups
   2. Push-ups
   3. Dips
Max out for 4 sets of above
exercises. Rest 3:00 in between
each rotation of all three exercises.

Back / Biceps
   Max pull-ups + 3 negs
   Wide pulldowns .... 3 x 15
   Reg. pulldowns .... 3 x 15
   Rev. pulldowns .... 3 x 15

Do 25 abs in between each set of
pulldowns

Cool down / Stretch

SATURDAY

Warmup/Stretch

CARDIO / LEG PT

Bike / leg PT / abs
Repeat 3 times:
   Bike 5:00
   Squats 1:00
   Lunges 1:00
   Calves 1:00
   Abs max 2:00
   (use dumbbells)

Sprints
   20m ....1/2 pace x 2
   20m ....full sprint x 3
   40m ....3/4 pace x 2
   40m ....full sprint x 3
   60m ....full sprint x 5
   80m ....full sprint x 3
   100m ....full sprint x 3
   (rest = walk back to starting line)

Cool down / Stretch

Week 5

Weights / PT / Cardio Mix

MONDAY

Warmup/Stretch

UPPER BODY

Push/Pull day
Repeat 10 times:
    Jumping jacks 10
    Push-ups 10

    Bench press .... 4 x 25 reps
    Crunches X 25 between bench
      press sets

Repeat 4 times:
    Pull-ups .... max
    Pulldowns 15
    Military press 15
    Pushdowns 15
    Dips .... max
    Abs of choice 50

Bike — lifecycle pyramid
    Levels 1-12-1 .... 1:00 each level
      (manual mode)
    Total time .... 23 minutes
    Push / pull peddle

TUESDAY

Warmup/Stretch

LOWER BODY

Repeat 5 times:
    Squats 40
    Lunges 20/leg
    Jog .... 1/8 mile in 1:00

    Swim with fins 1000m
    Swim without fins:
    Flutterkicks only 100m
    Arm pull only 100m
    Flutterlicks only 100m
    Over/unders 100m
    Cool down 100m

    Cool down / Stretch

WEDNESDAY

Warmup/Stretch

INTERVAL TRAINING
    50 yd sprint / jog/walk .. 30 minutes

Ab Workout #4
Repeat 2–4 times:
    Advanced Crunch 25
    Reverse crunch 25
    Advanced R/L crunch 25
    Advanced Reverse 25

Lower / Upper Back
    Lower Back Ex # 1 25
    Lower back Ex #2 25
    Swimmers 25
    Reverse push-ups 25
    Arm Haulers 25

THURSDAY

Warmup/Stretch

FULL BODY

Cool down / Stretch

25,20,15 circuit of reps
    (alternate each exercise)
Bench press 25, 20, 15
Military press 25, 20, 15
Squats w/ heel raises 25, 20, 15
Lunges 25, 20, 15
Pulldowns or ups 25, 20, 15
Leg ext 25, 20, 15
Pushdowns 25, 20, 15
Leg curls 25, 20, 15
Bicep curls 25, 20, 15
Tricep ext 25, 20, 15
Bent knee heel raise 25, 20, 15
L/R/reg./reverse crunches 25
Bike / jog 5:00

FRIDAY

Warmup/Stretch

DAY OFF - STRETCH

SATURDAY

Warmup/Stretch

FULL BODY MAX

    Bench .... max
    Squats .... max
    (work up to max in 5 sets)
    Rest 3:00 in between each set

    Incline bench 4x10
    Leg curls .... 4 x 20
    Leg ext .... 4 x 20

Pt max in 2:00 each:
    Max pull-ups ....
    Max push-ups ....
    Max situps ....
    Max dips ....

Sprint
    2 mile run .... timed
    500 yd swim .... timed

Weeks 6–8

Rest Week

Weights / PT / Cardio Mix

MONDAY

Warmup/Stretch
1 mile jog or 10:00 bike

UPPER BODY
Bench press 10, 8, 6, 4, 2, 1
increasing weight each set 25 abs
of choice in between each set

Repeat 4 times:
Pull-ups .... max
Dips .... max
push-ups .... max in 1:00

Pulldown super set
Regular pulldowns .... 3 x 15
Reverse pulldowns .... 3 x 15
Wide pulldowns .... 3 x 15
25 abs between sets .... 9 sets x 25

Repeat 4 times:
Incline Bench DB 15
Bench Flies 15
Push-ups 15
Upright rows 15
Lat. raises 15
Military press 15

Cool down / stretch

TUESDAY

Warmup/Stretch

LEG WORKOUT
Repeat 3 times:
Run 1 .... mile
Squats 30
Lunges .... 20 / leg
Heel raises 30

Love Handles
  repeat 3 times
Side Oblique .... 25 each side
Inner Thigh crunch .... 25 / side
Outer Thigh crunch .... 25 / side

Lower / Upper Back
Lower Back Ex #1 25
Lower back ex #2 25
Swimmers 25
Reverse push-ups 25
Arm Haulers 25

Cool down / Stretch

WEDNESDAY

Warmup/Stretch

RUN - SWIM - RUN
Run or bike 20:00
Swim .... 20:00 with fins
Run or bike 10:00

Ab workout #1
Repeat 4–5 times:
Reg. Crunches 25
Rev. Crunches 25
Alt. reg./rev. crunches .... 25 each
Left leg lever crunches 25
Right leg lever crunches 25

THURSDAY

Warmup/Stretch

UPPER BODY PULL
Max pull-ups +3 negatives
Wide pulldowns .... 3 x 15
Regular pulldowns .... 3 x 15
Reverse pulldowns .... 3 x 15

Bent over rows .... 3 x 10

Bicep curls 30
Hammer curls .... 30 / arm
Concentration curls 10
    (slow - 5 count curls)

Assisted pull-ups 100
    (do 100 reps in as few sets as
    possible)
Remember, keep your feet on the
ground when do these if you have
to. So as many deadhang pull-ups
as you can then resort to assisted.

FRIDAY

Warmup/Stretch

LEG SUPERSET
Repeat 2–3 times:
Squats .... 20 w/ weights
1/2 squats 20
4-count squats 10
Walking squat 10/side
Lunges 10-20/leg
Walking lunges .... 20 steps
Calves regular, toe in, toe out,
and bent knee (each) 20

Sprints (rest = walk to starting line)
10m .... sprint x 10
20m .... Sprint x 5
40m .... Sprint x 5
60m .... Sprint x 4
100m .... sprint x 3

Advanced Ab workout #2
Repeat 3–4 times
Situps 25
Cross situps .... 25 each side
Flutterkicks 50
Leg levers 50
V-ups 20
Atomic situps 20

SATURDAY

Warmup/Stretch

CHEST TRI, SHOULDERS
Bench press .... 5 x 5
Incline DB .... 3 x 15
Bench flies .... 3 x 15
Dips .... 3 x 15

Mega Shoulder workout x 2
W / 5 lbs DBs
and 2-3 lbs DBs
(non-stop)

Spartan run
Run .... 1 mile
Push-ups 100
Abs of choice 100
Run .... 1 mile
Push-ups 75
Abs of choice 75
Run .... 1 mile
Push-ups 50
Abs of choice 50

Cool down / Stretch

Weeks 10–12

Weights / PT / Cardio Mix

MONDAY

Warmup/Stretch

FULL BODY
Alternating circuit
Repeat 4 times:
Pulldowns 15
Crunches 25
Bench press 15
Crunches 25
Bike 4:00
Repeat 3 times:
Military 15
Squats w/heel raises 20
Lunges .... 15 /leg
Side crunches .... 25 / side
Bike 4:00
Bicep curls 15
Tricep ext 15
Leg ext 20
Leg curls 20
Bike 4:00

   Lifecycle pyramid
Level 1-12-1
1:00 each level (manual mode)
Total time .... 23 minutes

Cool down / Stretch

TUESDAY

Warmup/Stretch

SHOULDERS
Mega-shoulderworkout
  (1, 2 and 5 lbs DBs)
Lateral raises 10
Lat raises (thumb up) 10
Lat raise(thumb up/down) 10
Front raise (thumb up) 10
Front raise (thumb up/down) 10
Cross over jacks 10
Military press 10

Run .... 5 miles

Cool down / Stretch

WEDNESDAY

Warmup/Stretch

UPPER BODY WEIGHT / PT CIRCUIT
  (no rest)
Pull-ups .... max +3 negative
Dips .... max + 3 negatives
Abs .... max in 2:00
Bench press .... 50% max
  (max +3 negatives)
Push-ups .... max in 1:00
Pulldowns .... 50% bodyweight
  (max + 3 negatives)
Abs .... max in 2:00
Bicep curls .... max reps (10–20lbs)
Tri ext .... max reps (10–20lbs)
Abs .... max in 2:00

Swim sprints
Repeat 10 times
Sprint 100m
Slow (catch breath) 50m
Total 1500m

Cool down / Stretch

THURSDAY

Warmup/Stretch

LEGS AND LOVE HANDLE

Mega Circuit
  Repeat ten times:
  Jumping Jacks 10
  Squats 10

  Repeat 3-4 times:
  Squats .... 30 w/DB
  Lunges .... 15 / leg w/DB
  Calves .... 30 w/ DB
  Side Oblique .... 25 /side
  Inner Thigh crunch 25
  Outer Thigh crunch 25
  Leg ext 25
  Leg curls 25
  Squats .... 20 w/weight

No weight PT
  Squats 1:00
  Lunges 1:00
  calves 1:00

Cool down / Stretch

FRIDAY

Warmup/Stretch

Repeat 10–20 times:
Jumping jacks 10
Push-ups 10

Repeat 4 times:
Bench press 15
Pulldowns 15
Push-ups 25
Reverse push-ups 20
Pull-ups .... max
Dips .... max
Tricep ext 15
Reg./Rev. crunches 50
Lower back #1/2 25
Bicep curls 20
Hammer curls 20
Military press 15
Abs of choice 50

Repeat 2 times:
MegaShoulder Workout
use 5 lbs DBs and 2 lb DBs.

Cool down / Stretch

SATURDAY

Warmup/Stretch

LAST TRIATHLON OF THE YEAR

Run ....5 miles
Swim 1000m
Bike or run 30:00

Cool down / Stretch

Week 13

Loading Phase

MONDAY

CHEST / TRICEPS

Jog	1/4 mile
Stretch	10 minutes

Bench Press	10, 8, 6, 4, 2, 1 max (increasing weight each set)
Push-ups	2 sets max
Military Press	3 x 15
Dips	2 sets max

Superset:
4 sets each:

Crunches	25–40 reps (No rest)
1/2 situps	25–40 reps (No rest)

Run	2 miles

TUESDAY

BACK & BICEPS

Jog	1/4 mile
Stretch	10minutes

Pull-ups	2 sets max
Pulldowns	3 x 10
Rows	3 x 10
Curls	3 x 10 / arm
Bar Curls	3 x 10

Run	2 miles / Stretch

WEDNESDAY

LEGS

Jog	1/4 mile
Stretch	10minutes

Squats	3 x 15
Lunges	3 x 15 w/dumbells
Calf raises	3 x 15

Sprints:

	10 yd x 5
	20 yd x 5
	40 yd x 3
	100 yds x 2
	220 yds x 1

Swim with fins	30:00

THURSDAY

CHEST & BACK

Jog	1/4 mile
Stretch	10 minutes

Bench Press	5 x 5 (80% max)
Push-ups	2 x's max
Dips	2 sets max
Pull-ups	2 sets max
Pulldowns	3 x 10
Dumbell rows	3 x10
Curls	3 x 10 / arm
Bar Curls	3 x 10

Run	2 miles

FRIDAY

SHOULDERS

Jog	1/4 mile
Stretch	10minutes
Military	8 x 15 reps (30 second rest)
Dumbell PT	3x's
Reverse Flies	15
Upright Rows	15
Shrugs	15
Lateral raises	15
Tri Extension	15

Abs:

1/2 Situps	25
Leg levers	25
Left Situps	25
Right Situps	25
Run	2 miles

Mega Shoulder Workout
5 lbs, 2 lbs, 0 lbs

SATURDAY

LEGS

Jog	1/4 mile
Stretch	10minutes

Squats	3 x 20
Lunges	3 x 10
Calf raises	3 x 15

Sprints:

	10 yds x 5
	20 yds x 5
	40 yds x 3
	100 yds x 2
	220 yds x 1

Weeks 1–2

Loading Phase

<table>
<tr><td colspan="2">MONDAY</td></tr>
</table>

MONDAY

CHEST & BACK

Superset: 8 sets (no rest)
  Incline Dumbbell
  Bench Press .... 10–12 reps
  Reverse Pull-up .... 10–12 reps

Superset: 4 sets (no rest)
  Crunches .... 25–40 reps
  Leg Raises .... 25–40 reps

TUESDAY

SHOULDERS & ARMS

Superset: 8 sets
  Miltary press .... 10–12 reps
  Upright Rows .... 10–12 reps
  Dumbbell Curls .... 10–12 reps
  Triceps Extensions .... 10–12 reps

WEDNESDAY

LEGS

Stretch Superset: 8 sets (no rest)
  Lunges .... 10–12 reps
  Leg Curls .... 10–12 reps
  Calf Raises .... 10–12 reps

Superset: 4 sers (no rest)
  Squats .... 25 reps
  Side crunches .... 25 reps

THURSDAY

CHEST & BACK

Stretch

Superset: 8 sets (no rest)
  Incline Dumbbell
    Bench Press .... 10–12 reps
  Reverse Pull-up .... 10–12 reps

Superset: 4 sets (no rest)
  Crunches .... 25–40 reps
  Leg Raises .... 25–40 reps

FRIDAY

SHOULDERS & ARMS

Stretch Superset: 8 sets
  Upright Rows .... 10–12 reps
  Dumbbell Curls .... 10–12 reps
  Triceps Extensions .... 10–12 reps

SATURDAY

LEGS

Superset: 8 sets (No rest)
  Lunges .... 10–12 reps
  Leg Curls .... 10–12 reps
  Calf Raises .... 10–12 reps

Superset: 4 sets (No rest)
  Squats .... 25 reps
  Side crunches .... 25 reps

Week 3

Loading Phase

MONDAY

CHEST & BACK

Superset: 8 sets (No rest)
Incline Dumbbell .... 10–12 reps
Bench Press .... 10–12 reps
Reverse Pull-up .... 10–12 reps

Superset: 3 sets (No rest)
Dips .... 10–12 reps
Dumbbell Rows .... 10–12 reps

Superset: 5 sets (No rest)
Crunches .... 25–40 reps
Leg Raises .... 25–40 reps

TUESDAY

SHOULDERS & ARMS

Superset: 8 sets (1 minute rest)
Upright Rows .... 25–40 reps
Crunches .... 8 x 25
Reverse Fly (3 sets) .... 10–12 reps
    (1 minute rest)

Superset: 8 sets (No rest)
Dumbbell Curls .... 10–12 reps
Triceps Extensions........... 10–12 reps

Superset: 3 sets (No rest)
Triceps Extensions........... 10–12 reps
Biceps Curls .... 10–12 reps

WEDNESDAY

LEGS

Superset: 8 sets (No rest)
Lunges .... 10–12 reps
Leg Curls .... 10–12 reps

Superset: 3 sets (No rest)
Dumbbell Squats .... 10–12 reps
Leg Curls .... 10–12 reps

Superset: 9 sets (No rest)
Calf Raises .... 10–12 reps
Crunches .... 9 x 25

THURSDAY

CHEST & BACK

Superset: 8 sets (No rest)
Incline Dumbbell.............. 10–12 reps
Bench Press .... 10–12 reps
Reverse Pull-up .... 10–12 reps

Superset: 3 sets (No rest)
Dips .... 10–12 reps
Dumbbell Rows .... 10–12 reps

Superset: 5 sets (No rest)
Crunches .... 25–40 reps
Leg Raises .... 25–40 reps

FRIDAY

SHOULDERS & ARMS

Superset: 8 sets (1 minute rest)
Upright Rows .... 10–12 reps
Crunches .... 8 x 25
Reverse Fly (3 sets) .... 10–12 reps
    (1 minute rest)

Superset: 8 sets (No rest)
Dumbbell Curls .... 10–12 reps
Triceps Extensions........... 10–12 reps

Superset: 3 sets (No rest)
Triceps Extensions........... 10–12 reps
Biceps Curls .... 10–12 reps

SATURDAY

LEGS

Superset: 8 sets (No rest)
Lunges .... 10–12 reps
Leg Curls .... 10–12 reps

Superset: 3 sets (No rest)
Dumbbell Squats .... 10–12 reps
Leg Curls .... 10–12 reps

Superset: 9 sets (No rest)
Calf Raises .... 10–12 reps
Crunches .... 9 x 25

Week 4

Loading Phase

MONDAY

CHEST & BACK

Superset: 8 sets (No rest)
Incline Dumbbell .... 10–12 reps
Bench Press .... 10–12 reps
Reverse Pull-up .... 10–12 reps

Superset: 3 sets (No rest)
Dips .... 10–12 reps
Dumbbell Rows .... 10–12 reps

Superset: 6 sets (No rest)
Crunches .... 25–40 reps
Leg Raises .... 25–40 reps

Superset: 3 sets (No rest)
Flat Fly's .... 10–12 reps
Pulldowns .... 10–12 reps

TUESDAY

SHOULDERS & ARMS

Superset: 8 sets (1 minute rest)
Upright Rows .... 10–12 reps

Superset 3 sets (30 second rest)
Reverse Flys .... 10–12 reps
Military Press .... 10–12 reps

Superset: 8 sets (No rest)
Dumbbell Curls .... 10–12 reps
Triceps Ext .... 10–12 reps

Superset: 3 sets (No rest)
Dips .... 10–12 reps
Hammer Curls .... 10–12 reps

Superset: 3 sets
TricepsKickback .... 10–12 reps
Barbell Curls .... 10–12 reps

WEDNESDAY

LEGS

Superset: 8 sets (No rest)
Lunges .... 10–12 reps
Leg Curls .... 10–12 reps

Superset: 6 sets (No rest)
Dumbbell Squats .... 10–12 reps
Leg Curls .... 10–12 reps

Superset: 12 sets (No rest)
Calf Raises .... 10–12 reps
Crunches .... 12 x 25

THURSDAY

CHEST & BACK

Superset: 8 sets (No rest)
Incline Dumbbell .... 10–12 reps
Bench Press .... 10–12 reps
Reverse Pull-up .... 10–12 reps

Superset: 3 sets (No rest)
Dips .... 10–12 reps
Dumbbell Rows .... 10–12 reps

Superset: 6 sets (No rest)
Crunches .... 25–40 reps
Leg Raises .... 25–40 reps

Superset: 3 sets (No rest)
Flat Fly's .... 10–12 reps
Pulldowns .... 10–12 reps

FRIDAY

SHOULDERS & ARMS

Superset: 8 sets (1 minute rest)
Upright Rows .... 10–12 reps

Superset: 3 sets (30 second rest)
Reverse Flys .... 10–12 reps
Military Press .... 10–12 reps

Superset: 8 sets (No rest)
Dumbbell Curls .... 10–12 reps
Triceps Ext .... 10–12 reps

Superset: 3 sets (No rest)
Dips .... 10–12 reps
Hammer Curls .... 10–12 reps

Superset: 3 sets
Triceps Kickbacks .... 10–12 reps
Barbell Curls .... 10–12 reps

SATURDAY

LEGS

Superset: 8 sets (No rest)
Lunges .... 10–12 reps
Leg Curls .... 10–12 reps

Superset: 6 sets (No rest)
Dumbbell Squats .... 10–12 reps
Leg Curls .... 10–12 reps

Superset: 12 sets (No rest)
Calf Raises .... 10–12 reps
Crunches .... 12 x 25

Weeks 5

Growth Phase

MONDAY

CHEST & BACK

Repeat 4 times:
Dumbells Fly 10–12
  (60 seconds rest)
Barbell Rows 10–12
  (60 seconds rest)

Repeat 8 times:
Bench Press .... 4–7 reps
  (90 second rest)
Wide Pullup 4–7reps
  (90 second rest)

Repeat 3 times:
Incline Bench Press .... 4–7 reps
  (90 second rest)
Bent Over Rows .... 4–7 reps
  (90 second rest)

Repeat 4 times:
Crunches .... 40 reps
  (90 second rest)
Rev. Crunch .... 40 reps
  (90 second rest)

TUESDAY

SHOULDERS & ARMS

Repeat 5 times:
Upright Rows .... 4–7 reps
  (90 second rest)
Reverse Flys .... 4–7 reps
  (90 second rest)

Repeat 8 times:
Bicep Curls 4–7reps
  (90 second rest)
Triceps Ext .... 4–7 reps
  (90 second rest)

Repeat 5 times:
Side Crunches .... 40 each side
Leg lever crunch .... 40 each leg

WEDNESDAY

LEGS

Repeat 8 times:
Squats .... 4–7 reps
  (90 second rest)
Leg Curls................................ 4–7 reps
  (90 second rest)

Repeat 3 times:
Lunges .... 4–7 reps
  (90 second rest)
Leg Curls................................ 4–7 reps
  (90 second rest)

Repeat 6 times:
Calf Raise .... 4–7 reps
Leg Ext .... 4–7 reps

THURSDAY

CHEST & BACK

Repeat 4 times:
DumbellBench .... 10–12 reps
  (60 seconds rest)
Bentover Rows .... 10–12 reps
  (60 seconds rest)

Repeat 8 times:
Bench Press .... 4–7 reps
  (90 second rest)
Wide Pullup 4–7reps
  (90 second rest)

Repeat 3 times:
Incline Bench Press .... 4–7 reps
  (90 second rest)
Bent Over Rows .... 4–7 reps
  (90 second rest)

Repeat 4 times:
Crunches .... 40 reps
  (90 second rest)
Leg Raises .... 40 reps
  (90 second rest)

FRIDAY

SHOULDERS & ARMS

Repeat 5 times:
Upright Rows .... 4–7 reps
  (90 second rest)
Reverse Flys .... 4–7 reps
  (90 second rest)

Repeat 8 times:
Bicep Curls 4–7reps
  (90 second rest)
Triceps Ext .... 4–7 reps
  (90 second rest)

Repeat 5 times:
Side Crunches .... 40 each side
Leg lever crunch .... 40 each leg

SATURDAY

LEGS

Repeat 8 times:
Squats .... 4–7 reps
  (90 second rest)
Leg Curls................................ 4–7 reps
  (90 second rest)

Repeat 3 times:
Lunges .... 4–7 reps
  (90 second rest)
Leg Curls................................ 4–7 reps
  (90 second rest)

Repeat 6 times:
Calf Raise .... 4–7 reps
Leg Ext .... 4–7 reps

Weeks 6–8

Rest Week

Power Phase

MONDAY

CHEST & BACK

8 sets each:
  Bench Press .. 4, 4, 3, 3, 2, 2, 1, 1 reps
  (150 second rest)
  Pulldowns ..... 4, 4, 3, 3, 2, 2, 1, 1 reps
  (150 second rest)

Abs superset:
  Lower back / Upper Back Exercise
  Lower back Ex.#1 25
  Lower back ex. #2 25
  Swimmers 25
  Reverse push-ups 25
  Arm Haulers 25

Ab Workout #4
  Repeat 2–4 times:
  Advanced Crunch 25
  Cross-legged Reverse crunch 25
  Advanced R/L crunch ....25 each
  Advanced Reverse 25

TUESDAY

SHOULDERS & ARMS

4 sets of:
  Upright Rows .... 4, 3, 2, 1 reps
  (90 second rest)
  Reverse Flys .... 4–7 reps
  (90 second rest)
  Dumbbell Curls .... 4, 3, 2, 1 reps
  (120 second rest)
  Triceps Extensions....... 4, 3, 2, 1 reps
  (120 second rest)

Love Handles
  Repeat 3 times:
  Side Oblique .... 25 /side
  Inner-Outer Thigh crunch 25
  (both sides and legs = 100)

WEDNESDAY

LEGS

8 sets of:
  Squats .... 4, 4, 3, 3, 2, 2, 1, 1 reps
  (150 second rest)
  Leg Curls .... 4, 4, 3, 3, 2, 2, 1, 1 reps
  (150 second rest)

3 sets of:
  Calf Raises .... 4–7 reps
  (60 second rest)
  Leg Ext .... 4–7 reps
  (60 second rest)

THURSDAY

CHEST & BACK

8 sets of:
  Bench Press ... 4, 4, 3, 3, 2, 2, 1, 1 reps
  (150 second rest)
  Pulldowns ..... 4, 4, 3, 3, 2, 2, 1, 1 reps
  (150 second rest)

Abs superset:
  Lower back / Upper Back Exercise
  Lower back Ex.#1 25
  Lower back ex. #2 25
  Swimmers 25
  Reverse push-ups 25
  Arm Haulers 25

Ab Workout #4
  Repeat 2–4 times:
  Advanced Crunch 25
  Cross-legged Reverse crunch 25
  Advanced R/L crunch ....25 each
  Advanced Reverse 25

FRIDAY

SHOULDERS & ARMS

4 sets of:
  Upright Rows .... 4, 3, 2, 1 reps
  (90 second rest)
  Reverse Flys .... 4–7 reps
  (90 second rest)
  Dumbbell Curls .... 4, 3, 2, 1 reps
  (120 second rest)
  Triceps Extensions....... 4, 3, 2, 1 reps
  (120 second rest)

Love Handles
  Repeat 3 times:
  Side Oblique .... 25 /side
  Inner-Outer Thigh crunch 25
  (both sides and legs = 100)

SATURDAY

LEGS

8 sets of:
  Squats .... 4, 4, 3, 3, 2, 2, 1, 1 reps
  (150 second rest)
  Leg Curls .... 4, 4, 3, 3, 2, 2, 1, 1 reps
  (150 second rest)

3 sets of:
  Calf Raises .... 4–7 reps
  (60 second rest)
  Leg Ext .... 4–7 reps
  (60 second rest)

Weeks 10–12

Power Phase

MONDAY

FULL BODY CIRCUIT

25, 20, 15 circuit of reps
For three sets of each:
(alternate each exercise)

Bench press 25, 20, 15
Military press 25, 20, 15
Squats w/ heel raises 25, 20, 15
Lunges 25, 20, 15
Pulldowns or ups 25, 20, 15
Leg ext. 25, 20, 15
Pushdowns 25, 20, 15
Leg curls 25, 20, 15
Bicep curls 25, 20, 15
Tricep ext 25, 20, 15
Bent knee heel raise ... 25, 20, 15
L/R/reg../reverse crunches 25
Bike / jog 5:00

TUESDAY

RUN AND BIKE

Jog .... 30 minutes
Bike .... 30 minutes

WEDNESDAY

FULL BODY CIRCUIT

Alternating circuit
Repeat 4 times:
Pulldowns 15
Crunches 25
Bench press 15
Crunches 25
Bike 4:00

Repeat 3 times:
Military 15
Squats w/heel raises 20
Lunges .... 15 /leg
Side crunches .... 25 / side
Bike 4:00

Repeat 3 times;
Bicep curls 15
Tricep ext 15
Leg ext. 20
Leg curls 20
Bike 4:00

THURSDAY

SWIM AND BIKE

Swim with fins
With fins ....500 m
Without ....500 m
Stroke of choice ....500 m

Bike LifeCycle pyramid
Level 1-12-1
1:00 each level
(manual mode)
Total time .... 23 minutes

FRIDAY

UPPER BODY CIRCUIT

Upper body weight / PT Circuit
workout
(no rest) x 2
Pull-ups .... (max +3 negatives)
Dips .... (max + 3 negatives)
Abs .... max in 2:00
Bench press .... 50% max
(max +3 negatives)
Push-ups .... max in 1:00
Pulldowns .... 50% bodyweight
(max + 3 negatives)
Abs .... max in 2:00
Military press .... max reps
(dumbells 10–20lbs)
Bicep curls .... max reps (10–20lbs)
Tri ext .... max reps (10–20lbs)
Abs .... max in 2:00

SATURDAY

LEGS

Leg /Bike PT
Repeat 5 times (with weights):
Squats 1:00
Walking lunges 1:00
Calves 1:00
Bike 3:00

Week 13

Nutrition and Weight Management

FEATURING

M. Laurel Cutlip, RD, LD

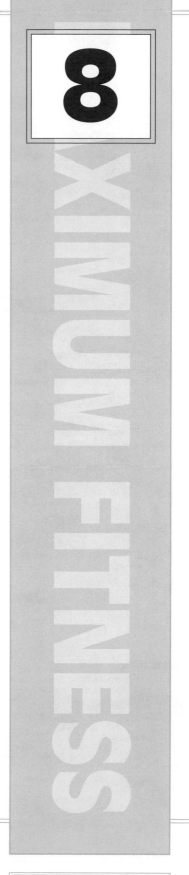

Did you know that drinking one can of soda each day can result in a 15-pound weight gain in a year? Are you currently using mayonnaise on your sandwiches? Change to mustard and you'll save your "buns" ten extra pounds. Small changes do make a big difference over the long term.

There is nothing magical about weight loss or gain. If there were, more than fifty percent of U. S. adults over age twenty wouldn't be overweight. The bottom line is calories eaten verses calories needed. Just as gas fuels our cars, calories fuel our bodies. At the gas station, we have four different fuel choices: diesel, low, mid and high octane. Calories, too, come from four substances in our food: proteins, carbohydrates, fats and alcohol. If your car has a 15-gallon tank, it doesn't matter whether you put in 16 gallons of cheap or expensive gas, it's going to spill out over your shoes. The same holds true for us. If we eat more calories than our bodies require, we gain weight, regardless of the calorie source. On the other hand, if we run out of gas, we use a can to fill our tank. If we consume fewer calories than we need, our bodies rely on our "internal gas cans," stored fat, and weight loss occurs.

Before we discuss building or battling the bulge, we should first review basic nutrition. What makes a healthy diet, you ask? Essentially, six nutrients are required for good health. These include water, carbohydrates, proteins, fats, vitamins and minerals.

Water

Water comprises about 75 percent of our total body weight and it serves many functions. Water helps regulate our body temperature. When we sweat, we rid ourselves of excess heat. Water serves as a transport medium, carrying needed nutrients to our cells and removing toxic substances and wastes. It cushions our body tissues and lubricates our joints. Water provides moisture for our respiratory system and is essential for our digestion. Since water is a major component of all cell structures, including muscle structure and function, it takes second place only to oxygen as the most important body component. Unfortunately, athletes often overlook this fact.

Improper fluid consumption during exercise can result in lack of coordination, irritability, fatigue, muscle cramping, mental confusion and more. Most adults need eight to nine cups daily; however, athletes require much more. To ensure sufficient fluid intake, the athlete should consume an additional 18 ounces 15 minutes prior to exercise and five ounces every 10 to 15 minutes thereafter. Beverages containing alcohol, coffee, tea and many colas are diuretics. They cause our kidneys to excrete more fluid than we normally would. Thus, plain water is the ideal hydration source.

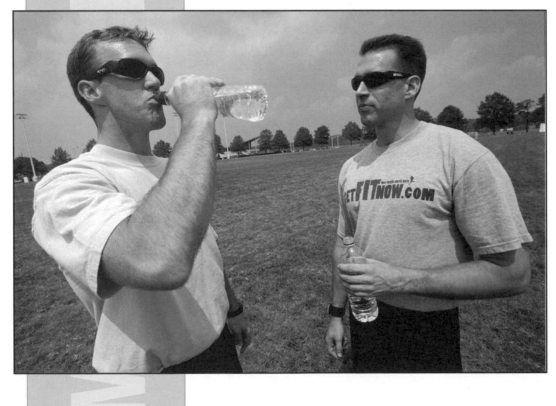

Carbohydrates

Since carbohydrates are the preferred source of energy for our muscles, they are extremely important to the athlete. Starch, sugar and fiber are all carbohydrates. Carbohydrate ingestion yields glucose, which enters your blood and is continuously withdrawn by your cells. It is the energy source they need to carry out their functions. Extra carbohydrate is converted into glycogen by your liver and is stored in your muscles and liver to be used as energy at a later time. Although some of our tissues can use other energy sources, your central nervous system depends on a continuous supply of glucose. When blood glucose levels fall, the liver reconverts stored glycogen to glucose. When stores are exhausted and replacement carbohydrates are not consumed, blood sugar again drops. This condition can lead to the breakdown of muscle, loss of sodium, dehydration, loss of consciousness and even death.

Fiber, an indigestible substance in plant-based food, may offer additional benefits. Fiber attracts water into the digestive tract, which softens the stools and prevents constipation. It also exercises digestive tract muscles to resist bulging and lessen the likelihood of diverticulosis. Because fiber causes waste products to pass through the intestines more quickly, it may decrease exposure time to potential cancer-causing agents. In the intestines, fiber binds with a small amount of fat, reducing the amount absorbed into the blood. This fat reduction may reduce your risk of developing artery and heart disease.

Carbohydrate intake should total about 60 percent of your daily calories; thus, a person consuming 2000 calories per day requires 300 grams. Recommended fiber intake is about 25 grams daily. Dried beans and peas as well as fruits, vegetables, breads, cereals and grains are outstanding carbohydrate sources. Go ahead, enjoy that pasta!

Proteins

Amino acids are the building blocks of protein. When they link together, protein is formed. Although protein can be used as an energy source, its major role is in building, repairing and maintaining body tissues. Protein is also necessary to manufacture enzymes, which are required for certain chemical reactions to occur in our bodies. Many people assume that, since muscles are made up of protein, the more protein they eat, the larger and stronger their muscles will be. This just isn't so. The avenue to increased muscle mass is exercise—use it or lose it! After your body utilizes the protein it needs to carry out its functions, excess amounts are converted to body fat. Protein is used as a fuel only if insufficient calories are consumed. In fact, excessively high protein intakes can be dangerous. This problem is explained further when we discuss common dieting myths.

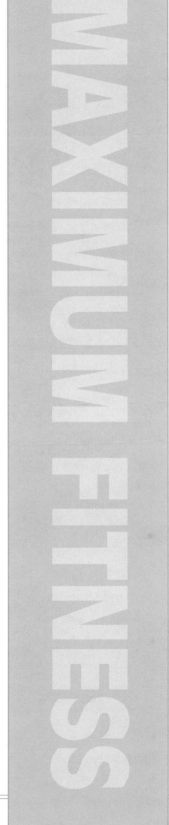

Protein-rich foods, such as lean meats, poultry, fish, tofu, cheese, milk, peanut butter, dried beans and peas are readily available in the United States. Most of us eat an enormous amount of this nutrient. The current recommendation of protein intake for most Americans is 0.8 grams per kilogram of body weight or about 0.364 grams per pound. This amount equates to 65 grams for a person weighing 180 pounds. A dinner consisting of a five-ounce chicken breast, eight ounces of skim milk, one cup of low fat macaroni and cheese along with one cup of broccoli provides enough protein for the entire day. Some athletes, such as competitive weight lifters, do have increased protein needs. Since their calorie requirements also climb, adequate protein is easily achieved when 15 to 20 percent of their total caloric intake comes from protein. The only thing you will gain from protein powders and supplements are unwanted pounds and an empty wallet.

Fats

We all have heard the horror stories about too much fat. Heart disease and certain cancers have been linked to high dietary fat intakes. We should, however, keep in mind that fat has very important functions in our bodies and that not all kinds of fat are created equal.

Only a limited amount of glycogen can be stored in our liver and muscles for energy. Fat storage capacity is endless; it is our energy reservoir. Once glycogen stores are depleted, the body must be fed or turn to its fat reserve to survive. Without fat, our bodies aren't able to absorb vitamins A, D, E, and K, which are fat-soluble. Like water, body fat assists us in maintaining proper body temperature. It protects our organs from heat and cold. Fat also cushions our organs, protecting us from mechanical shock.

Saturated fats, with the exception of coconut and palm oils, are solid at room temperature. These are our "bad fats." Some examples are fats in meat, cheese, whole milk and butter. "Good fats" include monounsaturated and polyunsaturated fats. They are liquid at room temperature and include all of the oils except those previously mentioned. Total fat should comprise no more than 30 percent of our total calorie intake, and less than 10 percent of fat calories should come from saturated sources. Since fat provides nine calories per gram, someone requiring 2000 calories daily should consume less than 65 grams of total fat. The saturated fat limit would be 20 grams.

MAXIMUM FITNESS

Vitamins

In the office, on the television, at the gym, almost anywhere you go, people are talking about them and spending a great amount of hard-earned cash on them. What are they? Vitamins! Each of the thirteen discovered vitamins is necessary for human survival. Protein, carbohydrate and fat digestion, absorption and metabolism could not occur without them. Insufficient amounts will compromise the health of offspring. Resistance to illness, concentration ability, and tissue health and growth will also be impaired. A lack of only one vitamin, over time, will result in death.

The *"if some is good, more is better"* philosophy does not hold true in the case of vitamins. In fact, consumption of high amounts can result in serious health complications. Even the water-soluble vitamins can have adverse effects. While it is nearly impossible to ingest toxic amounts of vitamins through food alone, it is quite easy to consume too much from supplements. Additionally, the body more easily absorbs vitamins in foods than those in pill form. Play it safe—save your money and *eat your vitamins!* Outlined below are the roles of specific vitamins, good food sources, adult daily requirements (non-pregnant, non-lactating) and signs of deficiency and toxicity.

VITAMIN A

FUNCTIONS .... prevents night blindness, keeps body tissues healthy, allows for normal bone and teeth growth

BEST FOOD SOURCES ... dark green leafy vegetables, red, orange or yellow vegetables and fruits, liver, eggs, fish oils, and fortified foods such as milk

REQUIREMENTS .... 800 to 1000 microgram retinol equivalents

DEFICIENCY .... poor night vision, increased risk of osteomalacia (soft bones), and osteoporosis

TOXICITY .... liver damage, bone abnormalities, headaches, double vision, hair loss, vomiting

VITAMIN D

FUNCTIONS .... promotes strong bones and teeth

BEST FOOD SOURCES ... eggs, cheese, sardines, fortified milk, cereals and margarine

REQUIREMENTS .... 5 to 10 micrograms

DEFICIENCY .... increased osteoporosis and osteomalacia risk

TOXICITY .... Weak muscles and bones, kidney stones and damage, excessive bleeding

VITAMIN E

FUNCTIONS .... helps form cell membranes, increases resistance to disease and possibly reduces the risk of certain cancers as well as heart disease

BEST FOOD SOURCES ... vegetable oils, seeds, nuts and wheat germ

REQUIREMENTS .... 8 to 10 mg alpha-tocopherol equivalents

DEFICIENCY .... abnormal nervous system functioning, premature very-low birthweight infants

TOXICITY .... unknown but very high amounts may interfere with the functioning of other nutrients

VITAMIN K

FUNCTIONS .... promotes normal blood clotting

BEST FOOD SOURCES ... green leafy vegetables

REQUIREMENTS .... 55 to 80 micrograms

DEFICIENCY .... abnormal blood clotting

TOXICITY .... none known

VITAMIN C

FUNCTIONS .... repairs damaged tissues, promotes wound healing, increases resistance to infection, maintains healthy gums, bones, and teeth

BEST FOOD SOURCES ... citrus fruits and juices, strawberries, tomatoes, potatoes and raw cabbage

REQUIREMENTS .... 60 milligrams

DEFICIENCY .... scurvy (symptoms may include bleeding, improper wound healing, loose teeth, and swollen gums)

TOXICITY .... gastrointestinal pain and diarrhea

VITAMIN B1 (THIAMIN)

FUNCTIONS .... carbohydrate metabolism

BEST FOOD SOURCES ... whole grains, nuts, peas, beans, pork, enriched breads and cereals

REQUIREMENTS .... 1 to 1.5 micrograms

DEFICIENCY .... weak muscles, nerve damage, fatigue

TOXICITY .... none known

VITAMIN B2 (RIBOFLAVIN)

FUNCTIONS .... energy release and cell repair

BEST FOOD SOURCES ... poultry, enriched breads, cereals and grains, as well as green leafy vegetables, organ meats, cheese, milk, and eggs

REQUIREMENTS .... 1.2 to 1.8 milligrams

DEFICIENCY .... sore red tongue, dry flaky skin, cataracts

TOXICITY .... none known

NIACIN (NICOTINIC ACID)

FUNCTIONS .... allows cells to use fuel and oxygen

BEST FOOD SOURCES ... meat, fish, poultry, nuts, legumes, enriched cereals and whole grains

REQUIREMENTS .... 13 to 20 milligrams

DEFICIENCY .... pellagra (symptoms may include dermatitis, diarrhea, and dementia)

TOXICITY .... in very high doses, flushed skin, possible liver damage, high blood sugar and stomach ulcers

VITAMIN B6 (PYRIDOXINE)

FUNCTIONS .... assists in protein and red blood cell formation, helps produce antibodies and hormones.

BEST FOOD SOURCES ... meat, chicken, fish, organ meats, nuts, legumes, and whole grains

REQUIREMENTS .... 1.5 to 2 milligrams

DEFICIENCY .... dermatitis, anemia, convulsions, and nausea

TOXICITY .... nerve damage

VITAMIN B1

VITAMIN B2

NIACIN

VITAMIN B6

FOLATE (FOLACIN OR FOLIC ACID)

FUNCTIONS .... produces DNA and RNA to make cells, helps make red blood cells

BEST FOOD SOURCES ... dark green leafy vegetables, orange juice, dried beans, liver, whole grain breads and cereals

REQUIREMENTS .... 180 to 200 micrograms

DEFICIENCY .... increased risk of spina bifida in offspring, weakness, irritability, sore red tongue, diarrhea, weight loss, anemia

TOXICITY .... can mask B12 deficiency, which if untreated, can cause permanent nerve damage

VITAMIN B12 (COBALAMIN)

FUNCTIONS .... assists in DNA, RNA and nerve formation, helps make red blood cells, facilitates energy metabolism

BEST FOOD SOURCES ... meat, poultry, fish, dairy products and fortified foods

REQUIREMENTS .... 2 micrograms

DEFICIENCY .... numb hands and feet, fatigue, anemia

TOXICITY .... none known

BIOTIN

FUNCTIONS .... assists in energy production

BEST FOOD SOURCES ... eggs, liver, dried beans, nuts, whole grains and cereals

REQUIREMENTS .... 30 to 100 micrograms

DEFICIENCY .... loss of appetite, fatigue, dry skin, heart abnormalities and depression

TOXICITY .... none known

PANTOTHENIC ACID

FUNCTIONS .... assists in energy production

BEST FOOD SOURCES ... meat, poultry, fish, whole grains and legumes

REQUIREMENTS .... 4 to 7 milligrams

DEFICIENCY .... numb hands and feet

TOXICITY .... diarrhea and water retention

Minerals

Minerals, which are classified into two groups (macrominerals and trace elements), are essential nutrients that cannot be made by the body. They, too, have many important functions. Minerals are needed to form bones, teeth and blood cells. Without them, muscles couldn't contract and nerve impulses couldn't transmit. They regulate the distribution of water in the body, maintain blood pH, and assist in many cellular reactions. These fifteen nutrients are indestructible and are required in only minute amounts. Overdoses can damage your heart, liver and kidneys. Although there are some instances where supplementation is indicated, you should fulfill mineral needs through food alone unless advised by your doctor. Described below are mineral functions, food sources, adult daily requirements (non-pregnant, non-lactating), and the results of deficiency and toxicity.

CALCIUM

FUNCTIONS	required for blood clotting, nerve, muscle and cell membrane functions, builds bone and teeth, promotes enzyme reactions
BEST FOOD SOURCES	dairy products, green leafy vegetables, tofu, almonds and legumes
REQUIREMENTS	800 to 1200 milligrams
DEFICIENCY	increases risk for osteoporosis
TOXICITY	kidney stones and damage, constipation

PHOSPHORUS

FUNCTIONS	promotes bone, teeth, DNA and RNA growth, assists in energy production
BEST FOOD SOURCES	meat, poultry, fish, eggs, legumes, nuts and breads
REQUIREMENTS	800 to 1200 milligrams
DEFICIENCY	bone loss, weakness, loss of appetite and pain
TOXICITY	decreases calcium levels in the blood leading to bone loss

MAGNESIUM

FUNCTIONS	component of bones and many enzymes, needed for energy production, muscle contractions, normal nerve and muscle cell functioning

MAXIMUM FITNESS

CALCIUM

PHOSPHORUS

MAGNESIUM

BEST FOOD SOURCES ... whole grains, legumes, nuts
REQUIREMENTS .... 280 to 400 milligrams
DEFICIENCY .... muscle tremors, poor coordination, nausea, weakness, convulsions and poor appetite
TOXICITY .... nausea, low blood pressure, heart abnormalities, vomiting

CHROMIUM

FUNCTIONS .... allows body to use glucose
BEST FOOD SOURCE ..... nuts, whole grains and meat
REQUIREMENTS .... 50 to 200 micrograms
DEFICIENCY .... nerve damage and high blood sugar
TOXICITY .... none known

COPPER

FUNCTIONS .... facilitates energy production, component of enzymes, helps form hemoglobin and connective tissue
BEST FOOD SOURCES ... fruits, vegetables, nuts, seeds, legumes, liver
REQUIREMENTS .... 1.5 to 3 milligrams
DEFICIENCY .... anemia
TOXICITY .... liver damage, coma, nausea, vomiting and diarrhea

FLOURIDE

FUNCTIONS .... prevents tooth decay, strengthens bones
BEST FOOD SOURCES ... sardines, salmon, fluoridated water and tea
REQUIREMENTS .... 1.5 to 4 milligrams
DEFICIENCY .... tooth decay
TOXICITY .... brittle bones, stained or mottled teeth

IODINE

FUNCTIONS .... forms hormones that regulate the rate of energy usage
BEST FOOD SOURCES ... seafood and table salt
REQUIREMENTS .... 150 micrograms
DEFICIENCY .... enlarged thyroid and weight gain
TOXICITY .... enlarged thyroid

IRON

FUNCTIONS .... component of hemoglobin that carries oxygen to the cells

BEST FOOD SOURCES ... meat, poultry, fish, legumes, green leafy vegetables, dried fruits and legumes

REQUIREMENTS .... 10 to 15 milligrams

DEFICIENCY .... infections, anemia and fatigue

TOXICITY .... poisons children and may lead to hemochromatosis, a serious disease in which too much iron is deposited in the body tissues.

MANGANESE

FUNCTIONS .... a component of enzymes involved in energy and protein metabolism

BEST FOOD SOURCES ... whole grain products, tea, fruits and vegetables

REQUIREMENTS .... 2 to 5 milligrams

DEFICIENCY .... rare

TOXICITY .... nerve damage

MOLYBDENUM

FUNCTIONS .... component of enzymes

BEST FOOD SOURCES ... organ meats, milk, legumes and whole grains

REQUIREMENTS .... 75 to 250 micrograms

DEFICIENCY .... rare

TOXICITY .... may interfere with copper use

SELENIUM

FUNCTIONS .... protects cells from damage, assists with cell growth

BEST FOOD SOURCES ... seafood, meats, grains and seeds

REQUIREMENTS .... 50 to 70 micrograms

DEFICIENCY .... may damage the heart

TOXICITY .... nerve damage, fatigue, irritability, nausea, vomiting, diarrhea, stomach pain

ZINC

FUNCTIONS .... needed for wound healing, growth, reproduction, carbohydrate, protein and alcohol metabolism, and the making of DNA and RNA

BEST FOOD SOURCES ... meat, liver, eggs, dairy, whole grains, legumes and oysters

REQUIREMENTS .... 12 to 15 milligrams

DEFICIENCY .... loss of taste, smell and appetite, reduced resistance to infection, scaly skin, growth retardation

TOXICITY .... interferes with copper absorption and immune functioning, reduces good blood cholesterol (HDL), upsets stomach and may cause nausea and vomiting

SODIUM

FUNCTIONS .... regulates fluids, blood pressure, nerve and muscle function

BEST FOOD SOURCES ... processed foods and table salt

REQUIREMENTS .... a minimum of 500 milligrams

DEFICIENCY .... muscle cramps, dizziness, nausea and fatigue

TOXICITY .... may cause high blood pressure

POTASSIUM

FUNCTIONS .... fluid and mineral balance, blood pressure regulation, nerve and muscle function

BEST FOOD SOURCES ... fruits, vegetables, poultry, meat and fish

REQUIREMENTS .... a minimum of 2000 milligrams

DEFICIENCY .... abnormal heartbeat, muscle paralysis, weakness, lethargy

TOXICITY .... heart abnormalities

CHLORIDE

FUNCTIONS .... component of stomach acid, regulates fluid balance

BEST FOOD SOURCES ... table salt

REQUIREMENTS .... a minimum of 750 milligrams

DEFICIENCY .... growth failure, behavioral and learning problems, poor appetite

TOXICITY .... may cause high blood pressure

Diet Evaluation

Since you now know which nutrients your body requires, you can determine if the foods you consume are fostering maximum nutrition. Use *The Food Guide Pyramid* to evaluate your diet. Begin by keeping a record of what and how much you currently eat for three to five days. If you hope to lose or gain weight, complete a more detailed record as discussed later in this chapter. Record the amounts eaten in cups (the size of a tennis ball), tablespoons (a heaping teaspoon) or ounces (three ounces of cooked meat, chicken or fish, are about the size of a deck of cards).

Next, determine your calorie needs. Women and older adults require about 1600 calories daily. Girls in their teens along with active women and the

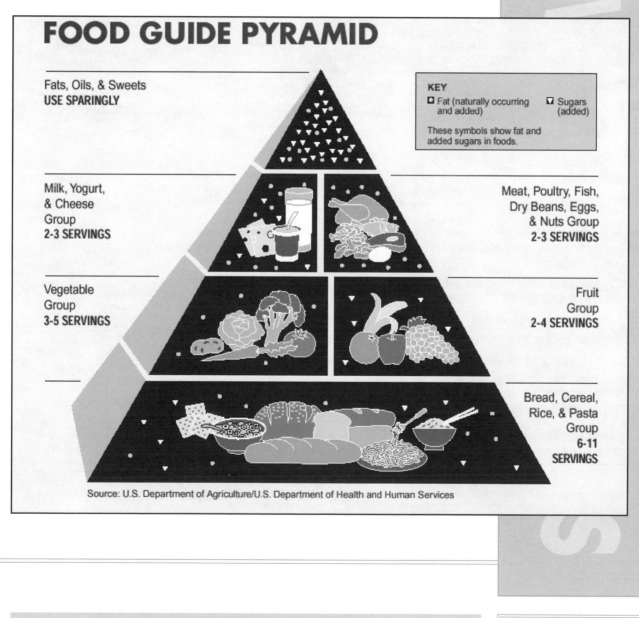

FOOD GUIDE PYRAMID

Fats, Oils, & Sweets
USE SPARINGLY

KEY
▽ Fat (naturally occurring and added)   ▽ Sugars (added)
These symbols show fat and added sugars in foods.

Milk, Yogurt, & Cheese Group
2-3 SERVINGS

Meat, Poultry, Fish, Dry Beans, Eggs, & Nuts Group
2-3 SERVINGS

Vegetable Group
3-5 SERVINGS

Fruit Group
2-4 SERVINGS

Bread, Cereal, Rice, & Pasta Group
6-11 SERVINGS

Source: U.S. Department of Agriculture/U.S. Department of Health and Human Services

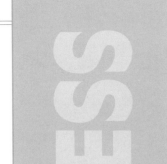

majority of men need approximately 2200 calories. Teen boys and active men require a daily caloric total of around 2800. Review the *"What counts as one serving?"* guidelines below to calculate how many servings you have consumed in each of the pyramid groups. How do your food choices compare to those recommended below? Now you can slowly adjust your food choices to coincide with those prescribed, and a healthy diet will result.

HOW TO USE THE FOOD GUIDE PYRAMID

What counts as a serving?	How many servings do you need each day?		
	1600 calories*	2200 calories*	2800 calories*
Bread, Cereal, Rice, and Pasta group • 1 slice of bread • About 1 cup of ready-to-eatcereal • 1/2 cup of cooked cereal, rice, or pasta	6	9	11
Vegetable Group • 1 cup of raw leafy vegetables • 1/2 cup of other vegetables—cooked or raw • 3/4 cup of vegetable juice	3	4	5
Fruit Group • 1 medium apple, banana, orange, pear • 1/2 cup of chopped, cooked, or canned fruit • 3/4 cup of fruit juice	2	3	4
Milk, Yogurt, and Cheese Group— preferably fat free or low fat • 1 cup of milk*** or yogurt • 1-1/2 ounces of natural cheese (such as Cheddar) • 2 ounces of processed cheese (such as American)	2 or 3**	2 or 3**	2 or 3**

Meat, Poultry, Fish, Dry Beans, Eggs, and Nuts Group—preferably lean or low fat
 • 2–3 ounces of cooked lean meat, pultry or fish
   These count as 1 ounce of meat:
   • 1/2 cup of cooked dry beans or tofu
   • 2-1/2 ounce soyburger
   • 1 egg
   • 2 tablespoons of peanut butter
   • 1/3 cup of nuts
	2 (5 oz. total)	2 (6 oz. total)	3 (7 oz. total)

*Recommended number of servings depends on oyour calorie needs:
• 1600 calories is about right for children ages 2 to 6 years,
• 2200 calories is about right for children over 6, teen girls, active women, and many sedentary men,
• 2800 calories is about right for teen boys and active men.

**Children and teens ages 9 to 18 years and adults over age 50 need 3 servings daily; others need 2 servings daily.

***This includes lactose-free and lactose-reduced milk products. Soy-based beverages with added calcium are an option for those who prefer a non-dairy source of calcium.

NOTE: Many of the serving sizes given above are smaller than those on the Nutrition Facts Label. For example, 1 serving of cooked cereal, rice, or pasta is 1 cup for the label, but only 1/2 cup for the Pyramid.

Weight Adjustment

Whether going on vacation, hosting a party or changing jobs, planning is essential. Weight loss or gain is no different. Altering your eating habits requires much effort. But, like most things in life, the greater the effort, the better the results. No single diet works for everyone.

Before attempting any dietary change, you must understand why it's important to you. To do this, I recommend you complete a weight loss (or gain) cost/benefit analysis. Compile a list of what you hope occurs as a result of your shaved or added pounds. This benefits list may include such outcomes as looking better, increasing athletic performance, improving your social life, finding clothes more easily, or increasing energy. Your second list should include all of the things you must give up or alter to achieve your goal, the cons. Planning meals, reducing your intake of favorite foods, feeling embarrassed around coworkers, and having less family time may be some of the sacrifices anticipated. Try not to overlook the importance of this step. Spend a lot of time on this task for it helps you identify your sources of motivation and the hurdles you will face. When completing this activity, remember that it's *your* list. Include only those items that are important to *you!*

Now it's time to perform the analysis. Review both lists to determine if the perceived benefits outweigh the costs. If so, perhaps you are ready for a behavior change and should proceed to the next step—self-evaluation. If the cost list is heavier, you may want to give yourself a specified period of time, a week or two, to attempt behavior change. Often positive change is a catalyst to further beneficial change and motivation builds. However, if after the trial period you discover you aren't ready, don't be too hard on yourself. Instead, defer your efforts to a time when you are able to make weight change a higher priority in your life.

Self-evaluation is next. Before you can make behavioral improvements, you first must learn what changes need to be made. Completing a detailed food journal, although time-consuming, will be extremely helpful. Construct a chart similar to the one below. Without altering your eating habits, record your behaviors over a course of three to five days. Be sure to include both weekdays and weekends.

DAY	TIME	FOOD CONSUMED	AMOUNT	WHERE	WITH WHOM	FEELINGS	CALORIES
Monday	8 AM	English muffin	1	home	alone	energetic	120
		grape jelly	1 tbsp				45
		orange juice	1/2 cup				60
	noon	Big Mac	1	McDonald's	Lillian	stressed	570
		french fries	large				400
		vanilla shake	regular				352
	4 PM	Coke	1 can	work	alone	tired	150
		chocolate cookies	4				400
	7 PM	boneless, skinless chicken	1 baked breast	home	alone	relaxed	142
		steamed green beans	1 cup				44
		white rice	1 cup				264
		water	1 cup				0

Nutrition Facts

Serving Size 1 cup (30g)
Servings Per Container About 19

Amount Per Serving	Team Cheerios	with 1/2 cup skim milk
Calories	120	160
Calories from Fat	10	10

	% Daily Value**	
Total Fat 1g*	**2%**	**2%**
Saturated Fat 0g	**0%**	**0%**
Polyunsaturated Fat 0g		
Monounsaturated Fat 0g		
Cholesterol 0mg	**0%**	**1%**
Sodium 210mg	**9%**	**11%**
Potassium 65mg	**2%**	**8%**
Total Carbohydrate 25g	**8%**	**10%**
Dietary Fiber 1g	**6%**	**6%**
Sugars 11g		
Other Carbohydrate 13g		
Protein 2g		

Vitamin A	10%	15%
Vitamin C	10%	10%
Calcium	10%	25%
Iron	25%	25%
Vitamin D	10%	25%
Thiamin	25%	30%
Riboflavin	25%	35%
Niacin	25%	25%
Vitamin B$_6$	25%	25%
Folic Acid	50%	50%
Vitamin B$_{12}$	25%	35%
Phosphorus	6%	20%
Zinc	25%	30%

* Amount in Cereal. A serving of cereal plus skim milk provides 1.5g total fat, less than 5mg cholesterol, 270mg sodium, 270mg potassium, 31g total carbohydrate (17g sugars) and 6g protein.
** Percent Daily Values are based on a 2,000 calorie diet. Your daily values may be higher or lower depending on your calorie needs:

	Calories:	2,000	2,500
Total Fat	Less than	65g	80g
Sat Fat	Less than	20g	25g
Cholesterol	Less than	300mg	300mg
Sodium	Less than	2,400mg	2,400mg
Potassium		3,500mg	3,500mg
Total Carbohydrate		300g	375g
Dietary Fiber		25g	30g

The calorie content of most foods can be found on their labels. Be sure to check the portion size. Calories listed are for the portion specified, so if the serving size listed is one cup and you consume two cups, you must double the calories. If you have a half-cup, the calories eaten are half those specified on the label. See the example below.

Food labels can be deceiving. Calories listed are for the food as packaged. If during preparation you add milk, margarine or any other ingredient, you must add the calories from these items as well. If there is no nutrition information on the label, your local library has numerous calorie books. Additionally, this information can be found on internet at www.caloriecontrol.org.

Weight Loss

Once you have completed your food journal, it's time to identify behaviors that can be improved. To estimate the number of calories you should consume daily to reach your desirable body weight, add a zero to the weight you would like to be. For example, an overweight person who wishes to weigh 150 pounds should attempt to consume approximately 1500 calories each day. Next, scrutinize the calories you are currently taking in. Are you consuming more than your estimated weight loss needs? How do your food choices coincide with those recommended on the food pyramid? Do you find that there is a particular time or day in which you consume more calories than at other times? Is overeating most likely to occur when you are with certain people or are at a specific place? Are you eating more when you are tired, bored, sad or stressed? Do certain foods or drinks account for a large percentage of your calorie totals? The following suggestions can help you combat problem behaviors.

If you find that you are taking in more calories than your weight loss needs require, identify those foods that contain the highest calories. Cut back on the portion size of these items and try to think of lower- calorie alternatives. If ice cream is a problem, for example, consider buying pre-portioned individual bars or cups. This way you won't be tempted to scoop out "just a little more." Possible substitutions for ice cream include juice bars, Italian ice, popsicles, fudgesicles and gelatin pops, all of which contain fewer calories. You might also consider purchasing these items in single servings at a restaurant or convenience store rather than keeping them in the house where they may tempt you.

If your food choices don't coincide with the food pyramid recommendations, don't try to change everything at once. Set a couple of mini-goals to move in the right direction. For example, if the guidelines suggest having four servings in the vegetable group and you are consuming two or less, make an effort to consume three each day. Once this change becomes routine, shoot for four. If over-consuming a particular group is the problem, slowly decrease the amount you eat. Remember, gradual change leads to long-term success.

If time of day triggers overeating, arrange to do something enjoyable during that period. Take a walk, call a friend, take a nap, visit the library, take a class, go to a movie or do anything to vary your routine. About 30 minutes prior to your problem time, eat a high fiber snack such as popcorn. Try not to let more than four hours pass between a meal or small snack during waking hours. You may be overeating because you simply are too hungry.

If you find that excessive eating occurs when you are with certain people or at a particular place, inform the others of your weight-loss efforts and ask for their support. Suggest getting together for a non-food-related activity. If you plan to join them for a meal, decide what you will eat before you reach the restaurant. Request that they help you stick with your decision. Ask family and friends not to offer you food and, if they still do, firmly say no. Eventually they'll get the message. If eating is associated with a particular activity, such as watching TV, resolve to eat in a different room and do nothing else while eating.

Before eating in response to emotional stress, remember that food is a temporary comfort, not a fix! Also, you will probably feel worse afterwards. Delay eating by five minutes and the urge may pass. Compile a list of alternative activities to be used during these situations. Taking a walk, calling a friend, reading a book or using relaxation techniques may help. Finally, realize that no one can make you feel inferior unless you let them.

Set yourself up for long-term success. Have healthy snacks on hand and decide what you will eat in advance. Keep problem foods out of the house and don't use the excuse that it's for company or the children. Shop from a list and go shopping only after you've eaten. Refrigerate leftovers after serving so they aren't easily available for seconds and always leave at least one bite on your plate to signify that you've had enough. Try to incorporate a change or two at a time rather than taking "the all or nothing" approach. Forgive yourself for slips—it's not what you do once in a while, it's what you do most of the while. As long as you don't give up, you will succeed. A child learning to walk falls a million times, and picks himself up another million. Eventually, he is walking and the falls become rare. Remember, it's progress, not perfection that is important. This weight didn't pop on in a week and it will not disappear in a week. Losing one-half to two pounds weekly is not only realistic, but it correlates best with keeping the weight off.

Popular Diets Analyzed

Not a magazine can be opened nor a bookstore browsed without your eyes being drawn to yet another recommended diet. Current diet book sales are estimated to exceed 140 million dollars yearly. Let's take a look at some of today's most popular regimens.

Just about everyone knows someone who has followed one of the numerous **low-carbohydrate, high-protein plans** currently being promoted. Initially they seem to work. Weight loss is quick the first week or two, but the loss is primarily water. When your body has exhausted its carbohydrate supply, it manufactures sugar from protein, including muscle protein. Your muscle tissue burns calories like crazy; fat burns hardly any at all. Because of the large amount of muscle loss, caloric needs decrease significantly; weight loss stops, and frustration sets in. When a normal diet is resumed, the pounds return. In many instances, you end up heavier than when the diet was initiated because your metabolic rate decreases along with your muscle loss.

Many low-carbohydrate, high-protein diet books encourage you to ignore recommendations from the American Heart, Dietetic, and Diabetes Associations as well as those of the United States Department of Agriculture. These authorities develop guidelines for optimal health based on extensive scientific research. Following low-carbohydrate, high-protein plans over the short term can result in bad breath, constipation, dizziness, irritability, improper kidney functioning, a loss of sodium and dehydration. Long-term effects may increase the risk for developing heart attacks, strokes and cancer.

Various **formula diets** have been around for years. Most of these do provide adequate nutrition with the exception of dietary fiber. Boredom, however, often sets in quickly and the formula loses its appeal. Since reasonable eating habits were not learned while consuming these low-calorie drinks, the weight is rapidly regained when the formula is abandoned.

Many theories lurk behind **high-fiber diets**. Fiber, when combined with water, causes bulk in the intestines and creates a feeling of fullness. Because most foods rich in fiber take a long time to chew, time available to eat a large quantity of food may be decreased. As a result, fewer calories are consumed. Generally, high fiber foods, such as fruits and vegetables, are low in calories and high in nutrition. Thus, most high-fiber diets are nutritionally sound. Just be sure you also eat adequate amounts of other foods. Let the food pyramid be your guide. Words of caution—don't increase your fiber too rapidly or constipation will set in, and make sure your water consumption rises simultaneously for the same reason.

The **Weight Watchers point and exchange systems** promote the intake of a variety of foods and are well balanced. Meal plans are individualized; weight-loss is slow, and behavior modification is taught. Many people also

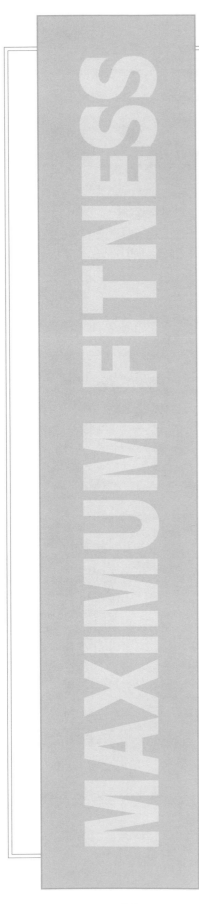

find the group support helpful. The cons include cost and time spent going to weekly meetings.

Protein powders for weight loss and gain will be discussed later in this chapter. Use the following section to assist you in evaluating specific diet plans.

Common Dieting Myths

Many fad diets promote quick weight loss but the loss is not primarily fat. It is chiefly a loss in water and muscle so that pounds return once a sensible diet is resumed. Identifying unsound claims is not easy. However, if it sounds too good to be true, it probably is! If the plan includes one or more of the following claims, be wary.

1. **A quick weight loss of five or more pounds weekly**. To lose five pounds in a week you would essentially need to fast. Furthermore, the loss would be primarily water, and weight loss would slow after the first week.

2. **Limited food choices**. Not only do these plans fail to meet your nutrient needs, they also foster boredom and the diet quickly gets discarded.

3. **Claims that one food will destroy the calories in another**. This claim is ridiculous; a calorie is a calorie!

4. **Promises little or no effort involved**. If this were true, no one would have a weight problem.

5. **Boasts that it has been suppressed by the medical profession**. There are few conspiracies in science. If you discovered the "fountain of thinness," don't you think the world would be talking about it?

6. **Requires you purchase special pills such as vitamin or mineral supplements**. In some cases, supplements are wise to ensure adequate nutrient intake. Most people, however, can get what they need following a healthy weight-loss plan.

7. **Statements that the diet is revolutionary**. If this were true, you would hear of its potential from scientific researchers while it was being tested.

8. **Promises improved beauty, strength or sexual performance**. Now really!

Gaining Weight

INSTEAD OF	HAVE	CALORIE SAVINGS
2% milk	nonfat milk	30 per cup
regular Italian salad dressing	fat free Italian	105 per 2 tbsp
American Cheese	part skim mozzarella	35 per oz.
raisin bran cereal	bran flakes	42 per 1½ cups
5 Ritz cheese crackers	15 Xtra cheddar Goldfish	30
2 Oreo cookies	12 chocolate Teddy Grahams	30
regular margarine	lite margarine	50 per tbsp
lemonade	diet lemonade	75 per cup
can of Coke	can of Diet Coke	150
hogie roll	hot dog roll	285
bagel	English muffin	150
mayonnaise	mustard	100 per tbsp
Whopper	Whopper Jr.	318
KFC biscuit	mashed potatoes and gravy	207
Big Mac	cheeseburger	252
Wendy's Frosty	McDonald's cone	215
1 cup of premium ice cream	1 popsickle	490
3 inch sausage patty	2 slices of bacon	160
potato chips	pretzels	54 per 1½ oz.
fruit pastry	toast with jam	230
peanut butter	light cream cheese	40 per tbsp
slice meat pizza	slice cheese pizza	40
croissant	dinner roll	95
cream-based soup	broth-based soup	80 per cup
prime rib steak	tenderloin steak	112 per 3½ oz.
6 buffalo wings w/dip	1½ cups chili	155
club sandwich	turkey sandwich	366
taco salad	2 slices cheese pizza	400
french fries	mashed potatoes	220

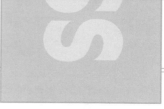

If you are on the thin side, you won't get much sympathy from family and friends. Many people fail to realize that gaining weight is just as difficult as losing it. Those desperate to bulk up often turn to protein powders. These are not the answer. Muscles become larger in response to one thing only—muscle use! Remember, excess dietary protein is converted to fat. Furthermore, when protein is broken down in the body, urea nitrogen, a waste product, is formed. A significant amount of water is needed to eliminate this waste and dehydration can result. This condition is detrimental to both health and performance. To gain muscle, your should be eating foods that give you adequate calories and nutrients, allowing you to workout even harder.

To get started on weight gain, first you need to determine how many calories you are currently taking in. Keep a detailed food journal. After calculating your average calorie intake, try consuming 500 to 1000 calories more each day. Theoretically, you should gain one to two pounds each week.

Athletes require additional amounts of all six essential nutrients, and food choices should be varied to meet these needs. Choose foods in accordance with the food pyramid plan. By using your calculated weight-gain calorie goals to choose foods in accordance with the food pyramid, you will consume adequate nutrients, including protein. If you find it difficult to eat more, the following suggestions will help.

Snack throughout the day instead of eating only three meals. Choose snacks that have lots of calories in a small volume. Dried fruits, juices, seeds and nuts are excellent examples. Use less water when preparing powdered drinks and consume only beverages that contain calories. Drink them through a straw because studies have shown that people actually drink more when using a straw. Keep food like raisins, which you would normally store in a cabinet, out in the open around your home and office. As you pass them by, take a handful. These items also can be kept in the car for frequent snacks. Eat larger portions at meals. For example, make sandwiches a little thicker. When preparing hot beverages, cereals and soups, use milk instead of water. Enrich the foods you currently eat by incorporating the suggestions below and remember, every little bite counts!

Additive Chart

ITEM TO ADD	FOODS TO ENRICH	CALORIE INCREASE PER TABLE
honey	canned fruit juice frozen desserts yogurt breads hot cereals	65
nonfat dry milk	fluid milk sauces soups casseroles puddings cottage cheese hot cereals	15
Karo syrup	canned fruit hot cereals yogurt	60
maple syrup	pancakes baked beans frozen desserts nuts	50
grated parmesan cheese	casseroles soups breads salads sauces vegetables hot cereals	25
canola or olive oil	sauces breads soups casseroles vegetables	120
sunflower seeds	salads cereals vegetables breads	50
raisins	cereals salads rice couscous	45
wheat germ	cereals casseroles salads	25

Weight Adjustment Supplements: Fact Vs. Whacked

"Lose weight while you sleep." "Eat all you want and watch the fat fall off." "This pill will make you look like you've been working out for years." "Flush fat out of the body." We've all seen the enticing ads. Weight loss and gain supplements, potions, and gadgets are now almost as popular as diet books, but do they work? Time to separate the "fat from the skinny."

The Food and Drug Administration now ban over 100 ingredients previously found in over-the-counter diet products from the marketplace because they failed to induce weight loss or suppress the appetite. Although ineffective for weight loss, supplements including spirulina (a type of blue-green algae), lecithin, starch blockers, fat blockers, magnet pills, glucommannan, skin diet patches, and coenzyme Q10 do promote a big, fat cash loss! Let's explore a few other substances in greater detail.

You name it, **kombucha tea** is claimed to cure it. In addition to burning body fat, this product is said to cure AIDS, cancer and so on. Not only is this product ineffective, it might be dangerous. Claims of liver damage, allergic reactions, drug interactions and death have been reported. **Ephedra**, also known as ephedrine, pseudoephrine, ma huang and epitonin, is another potentially fatal ingredient in weight-loss supplements. It can raise blood pressure, injure muscles, and induce nerve damage, psychosis, memory loss and stroke. It also has been linked to several deaths. **Carnitine** is a substance produced by the body. Consuming more via supplements does not improve athletic endurance or improve fat burning ability.

Product marketers suggest **chromium picolinate** builds muscle and helps you lose weight. The truth is that the claims haven't panned out in the research lab. Furthermore, since chromium is indestructible by the body, excess ingestion may have serious health risks.

Amino acids and protein powders have been marketed as a cure for obesity, insomnia, pain and depression. More often though, they have been pushed as muscle builders. As stated earlier, an overabundance of protein doesn't magically build muscle. Excess protein, in fact, is converted to body fat. So, not only will you fail to lose weight or gain muscle, you probably will gain fat.

Creatine is one of the most popular amino acid supplements. This one is said to enhance athletic performance but has failed to show its effectiveness outside of the laboratory setting. Gastrointestinal disturbances and muscle cramping have been reported, but how creatine will affect the body's organ systems over time is of greater concern. The expense of using weight adjustment supplements, in terms of your health and money, far outweighs any unlikely beneficial effects.

Before popping a pill or potion in search of an easy dietary fix, think hard. The "magic pill" isn't in the bottle; it's in the kitchen and gym. Boring as it may sound, eat reasonably, exercise hard and your goals will be achieved. For additional support or to find a qualified nutritionist in your area, contact The American Dietetic Association at www.eatright.org or 1-800-877-1600.

MAXIMUM FITNESS

Supplemental Schedule for Busy Weeks & Months

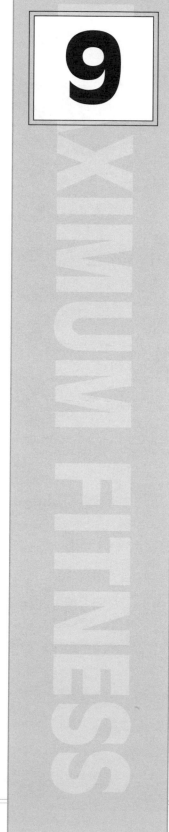

There will be times when it is impossible to exercise with such intensity year round. Illness, job and family requirements, and other factors prevent us from dedicating the several hours of exercise a week required in this book. Therefore, I have created a simplified plan for clients who travel frequently and cannot maintain these workouts at least one week every month. This program, which I have entitled *The Time Saver Workout*, is a combination of the fastest routines in the 52-week workout. This program is designed for people who have limited time to exercise (30 minutes a day maximum). These workouts can be expanded to accommodate your available workout time. If you only have time for ten minutes a day of exercise, use that time to stretch before you get into bed at night. Use your imagination—you would be surprised what can be done with a playground, hotel pool, pair of dumbbells, and a stationary bike.

At home/hotel room (no equipment)

10-Minute Workout (Repeat 5–10 times)
Jumping Jacks .... 10 reps
Push-ups .... 10 reps
Jumping Jacks .... 10 reps
Squats .... 10 reps

Minimal equipment (treadmill or bike)

Bike/Leg PT .... repeat three times
Squats .... one minute
Lunges .... one minute
Heel Raises .... one minute
Abdominal Exercise of Choice .... one minute
Bike .... four minutes

Weight machines (and dumbbells)

Mega-Shoulder Workout .... (two to five pound weights)
Full Body Circuit .... 18 minutes
Unlimited Ideas .... (use portions of book)

Full Body Workout

Repeat three to four times
Squats .... 20 reps
Lunges .... 20 reps
Calf Raise .... 25 reps
Crunches .... 50 reps
Push-ups .... 20 reps
Bench Dips .... 20 reps
Pull-ups .... MAX (playground, gym doors)

Spartan Run (Treadmill)

Repeat three to four times
Push-ups .... 50 reps
Crunches .... 50 reps
Run .... five minutes

A Final Note

It is never too late to begin a program of flexibility and exercise. The benefits of starting and continuing a fitness program will reward you throughout your life. In fact, studies by the Center for Disease Control and the Surgeon General have proven that the ONLY way to prevent heart disease, osteoporosis, and other degenerative diseases is to eat a well-balanced diet and exercise a minimum of 30 minutes at least five times a week.

Success depends on your readiness to change your sedentary lifestyle. Statistics suggest most people are not ready to change, accounting for a 50 percent dropout rate from exercising programs. What will motivate America to exercise? Perhaps knowing that an active lifestyle now will help you live longer and see your grandchildren have children. Maybe understanding the proper way to exercise will persuade you to begin a program. Or possibly seeing your children follow in your footsteps and never begin an active lifestyle will convince you. I wish I had the answer. You will have to find your own motivation to exercise. However, I am always available online to answer any questions at www.getfitnow.com.

Those of you who make fitness an important part of your lives, try to encourage a friend or family member to join you. Save someone you love from an inactive lifestyle and buy this book for them. You will be amazed at what a year of exercise will do to their life. I promise this book will change lives if you follow the workout as close as possible. Good luck and I hope this will be the best workout you have ever used.

To Your Health,
Stew Smith

Destination Cure

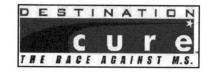

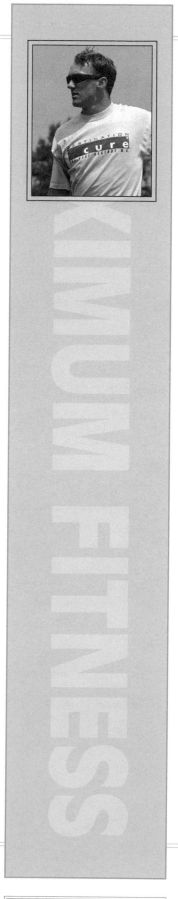

A portion of the proceeds from this book will be donated to Destination Cure, a non-profit organization dedicated to the long-term effort to raise public awareness and funds for researching a cure for Multiple Sclerosis (MS). MS is a neurological disease affecting nearly a million Americans, most of whom are stricken in the prime of their lives. The majority of Destination Cure's fundraising takes place at athletic competitions, and 100 percent of all funds raised go directly to MS research. For more information about Destination Cure please visit their web site at www.destinationcure.com

John Guandolo, the Founder of Destination Cure, is a native of Rockville, Maryland and a 1989 graduate of the U.S. Naval Academy in Annapolis, Maryland. Commissioned as a 2nd Lieutenant in the United States Marine Corps, Mr. Guandolo served as a platoon commander with an infantry battalion during Operation Desert Storm in Kuwait. After spending nearly five years in 2d Force Reconnaissance Company, Mr. Guandolo left the Marines and is now a Special Agent in the Washington Field Office of the Federal Bureau of Investigation. Mr. Guandolo is a nationally certified Paramedic and First Aid/ CPR Instructor, and volunteers for a local rescue squad, the American Red Cross, and the National MS Society in Washington, D.C.. John's motivation for Destination Cure comes from his mother, who has had multiple sclerosis since he was two years old. After years of witnessing her continued motivation and struggles, he sees this as an opportunity to make a difference. He dedicates his mission to her.

Frequently Asked Questions

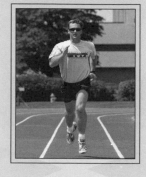

How Can I Run Faster?

As a fitness advisor for www.getfitnow.com, I have received numerous e-mails requesting workouts for the Marine Corps and Army's two- and three-mile PFT runs, in addition to programs for runners competing in 5K and 10K weekend races. The training philosophy for these distances are relatively the same—short distance, faster pace.

The four-mile track workout has used interval training to improve the times of military and short-distance runners for years. Interval training is running at a specified pace for a particular distance, then increasing the pace the next distance. The four-mile track workout is broken into quarter-mile sprints and jogs, and one-eighth mile sprints and jogs for a total of four miles.

Four-Mile Track Workout

Jog for one mile in 7:00 - 8:00

Three sets of:	Sprint for a quarter-mile
	Jog for a quarter-mile in 1:45
Six sets of:	Sprint for one-eight mile
	Jog for one-eight mile in 1:00

Repeats

Another good speed workout is REPEATS. Simply run a certain distance as fast as you can a specified number of times. During this workout, you can slow to a walking pace to recover and catch your breath between sprints. Try one of the following distances for a challenging workout:

1 Mile Repeats:	1 mile x 3–4 (walk 1/2 mile in between) = 3–4 miles
1/2 Mile Repeats:	1/2 mile x 6 (walk 1/4 mile in between) = 3 miles
1/4 Mile Repeats:	1/2 mile x 12 (walk 1/8 mile in between) = 3 miles
1/8 Mile Repeats:	1/8 mile x 16 (walk 100 yards in between) = 2 miles

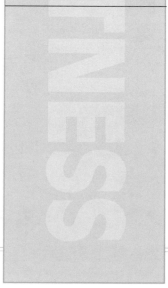

Avoid slowing to a walking pace to rest. The only rest during this workout is slowing to a jogging pace. Try to catch your breath while you jog.

MAXIMUM FITNESS

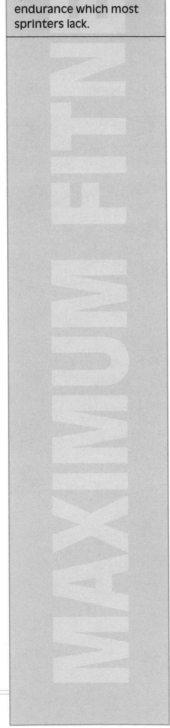

Sprint/Jogs

Finally, try incorporating shorter jogs with sprints for an extended period of time. This type of training builds the speed and endurance needed for PFTs, 5K and 10K races. Run approximately 50 yards as fast as you can, then jog 50 yards at a slower pace to catch your breath. I prefer to do this workout near telephone poles so I can sprint to one pole and jog to the next.

Sprint/Jogs
50-yard sprint/50-yard jog (for 10, 20, or 30 minutes)

How Can I Ace Any Military or Government Physical Fitness Test (PFT)?

Every six months, military personnel line up to take their physical fitness tests (PFT). Though each service differs in testing exercises and measuring criteria, most military personnel worry for several weeks prior to this event. However, for those who properly prepare themselves, the PFT can be just another workout.

Here are each service's PFT exercises and helpful tips to increase your overall score on test day:

TEST YOURSELF—The anxiety felt during these tests is primarily due to performing within a time limit. By timing your workouts, you grow accustom to "pacing" yourself, thus eliminating most anxiety.

PULL-UPS—During the pull-up and push-up test, perform as many as possible while adhering to proper form and technique. Look straight up at the sky to target your back muscles.

Recommended workout: The pyramid workout. Begin with one pull-up for the first set, two pull-ups for the second set, and continue to climb the pyramid until you have reached your maximum. Then, descend the pyramid until you are back to one pull-up.

PUSH-UPS—The wrong hand positioning can severely effect your maximum score. The perfect location for your hands is just outside shoulder width—enabling the chest, shoulders, and triceps to be equally taxed. Keep your hands at shoulder-height in the raised position. Your push-ups will weakened if your hands are too low, wide, close, or high.

Recommended workout: Try five sets of maximum push-ups in five one-minute periods.

CURL-UPS (SITUPS)–Pace is very important with this exercise. Most people burn out in the first 30 seconds with 30 curl-ups accomplished, only able to perform another 20 curl-ups within the next minute and a half. By setting a pace at 20 situps every 30 seconds, for instance, you can turn your score of 50 to 80 with very little effort.

Recommended workout: Try timing five 30-second sets, with setting your pace as your goal. A good pace is 20 situps in 30 seconds—totaling 80 situps in two minutes.

TIMED RUN–The most important thing is to not accelerate too quickly. Learn your pace and use it to set your goal to the finish. For instance, if your goal is to run the two-miles in 14 minutes, you must run a seven-minute mile or a one and a three-quarter quarter-mile.

Recommended workout: You can decrease your run time by running quarter-mile distances at your desired goal pace. Run quarter-mile repeats with 30 to 45 seconds rest periods for the distance of your PFT.

Remember to take big deep breaths, relax your upper body, and slightly bend your arms. Do not run flat-footed. Your heel should contact the ground first, then roll across your foot to your toe—heel-toe contact.

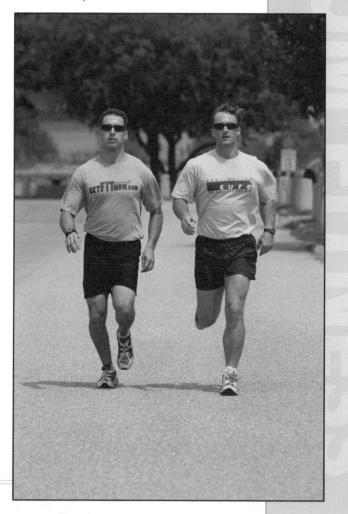

Meet the Authors

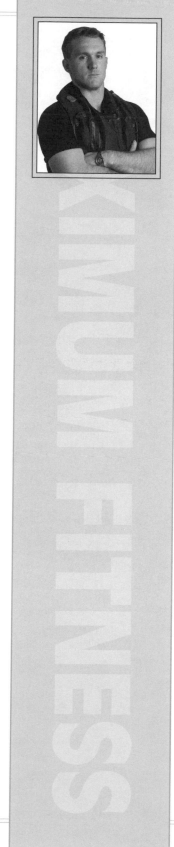

STEWART SMITH is a United States Naval Academy graduate and former lieutenant in the Navy SEAL Teams. During his four years on the SEALs Team, Stew learned to achieve maximum levels of physical fitness thanks to the knowledge of several Chief Petty Officer SEALS, Navy doctors and nutritionists. He later worked in the US Naval Academy Physical Education Department as the "personal trainer" to more than 4,000 Midshipmen. His four years in the Naval Academy and five years on the SEAL teams have enabled him to learn and perfect his unique techniques of rigorous, physical training.

Over half of Stew Smith's life has been devoted to athletics and exercise. His superior and exciting fitness methods have ranked him as one of the top military/fitness trainers in the country. He has a weekly fitness column on the military.com web site and is the author of numerous titles including **The Complete Guide To Navy SEAL Fitness** and **The TV Watchers Workout**. He is also the co-author of **The Boot Camp Workout** and the revolutionary and soon to be released **Combat Fat**. Stew's vast experience and love of fitness has compelled him to help others attain a goal of lifelong fitness.

Contributing Authors

JAMES VILLEPIGUE is certified by the International Sports Sciences Association (ISSA) and the Aerobics and Fitness Associations of America (AFAA) as a personal fitness trainer/counselor and weight room certified trainer. Throughout his career, James has passionately kept up to date with the latest trends and rapid changes within the bodybuilding and fitness world. The fact that James spend much of his childhood and adolescence overweight, combined with his ability to create success from his struggles, led him to dedicate his life to helping others make their fitness dreams and goals come true.

James has been a strength and conditioning coach for the United States Karate Team, a fitness advisor/moderator for www.getfitnow.com, and a

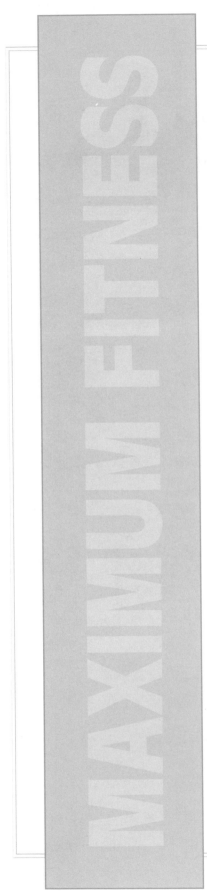

massage therapist. He is also the author of the upcoming books *The Body Sculpting Bible for Woman* and *The Body Sculpting Bible for Men*, and co-author of *Combat Fat*.

• • •

Upon graduating with honors from the University of Maryland, **M. LAUREL CUTLIP** completed a dietetic internship at the University of Virginia Medical Center. She became a health analyst for *Prevention* magazine and managing editor for *The Vitamin A+ Sieve*. Later, serving as an U.S. naval officer, "Laurie" counseled Naval Academy athletes on sports nutrition. She was both head of nutrition education and clinical dietetics at the National Naval Medical Center. Laurie, a registered dietician, now owns a private practice in Maryland where she lives with her husband Bob and two children, Matthew and Brenna.

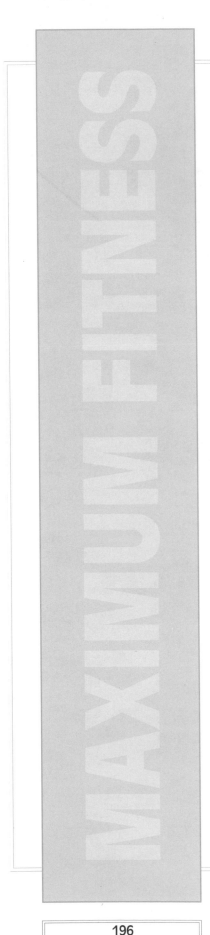